Is Human Embryo Experimentation Ethical?

Bonnie Szumski and Jill Karson

INCONTROVERSY

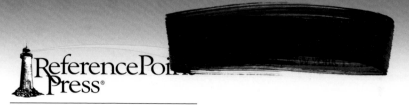

ReferencePoint
Press®

San Diego, CA

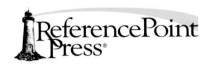

About the Authors
Bonnie Szumski has been an editor and author of nonfiction books for 25 years. Jill Karson has been an editor and author of nonfiction books for young adults for 15 years.

© 2013 ReferencePoint Press, Inc.
Printed in the United States

For more information, contact:
ReferencePoint Press, Inc.
PO Box 27779
San Diego, CA 92198
www. ReferencePointPress.com

Picture credits:
© Carlos Avila Gonzalez/San Francisco Chronical/Corbis: 38
© BSIP/Corbis: 59
© Owen Franken/Corbis: 64
© Brookes Kraft/Corbis: 75
© Photo Researchers, Inc: 7, 13, 29, 34
© Ron Sachs/CNP/Corbis: 22
© Paul Sakuma/Corbis: 78
Science Photo Library: 52
© Solvin Zankl/Corbis: 44

LIBRARY OF CONGRESS CATALOGING-IN-PUBLICATION DATA

Szumski, Bonnie, 1958-
    Is human embryo experimentation ethical? / by Bonnie Szumski and Jill Karson.
        p. cm. -- (In controversy series)
    Includes bibliographical references and index.
    ISBN 978-1-60152-456-0 (hardback) -- ISBN 1-60152-456-0 (hardback)
    1. Embryonic stem cells--Research. 2. Embryonic stem cells--Research--Moral and ethical aspects.
    3. Human experimentation in medicine--Moral and ethical aspects. I. Karson, Jill. II. Title.
    QH588.S83S98   2013
    174.2'8--dc23
                                                                    2012020155

Contents

Foreword

In 2008, as the US economy and economies worldwide were falling into the worst recession since the Great Depression, most Americans had difficulty comprehending the complexity, magnitude, and scope of what was happening. As is often the case with a complex, controversial issue such as this historic global economic recession, looking at the problem as a whole can be overwhelming and often does not lead to understanding. One way to better comprehend such a large issue or event is to break it into smaller parts. The intricacies of global economic recession may be difficult to understand, but one can gain insight by instead beginning with an individual contributing factor, such as the real estate market. When examined through a narrower lens, complex issues become clearer and easier to evaluate.

This is the idea behind ReferencePoint Press's *In Controversy* series. The series examines the complex, controversial issues of the day by breaking them into smaller pieces. Rather than looking at the stem cell research debate as a whole, a title would examine an important aspect of the debate such as *Is Stem Cell Research Necessary?* or *Is Embryonic Stem Cell Research Ethical?* By studying the central issues of the debate individually, researchers gain a more solid and focused understanding of the topic as a whole.

Each book in the series provides a clear, insightful discussion of the issues, integrating facts and a variety of contrasting opinions for a solid, balanced perspective. Personal accounts and direct quotes from academic and professional experts, advocacy groups, politicians, and others enhance the narrative. Sidebars add depth to the discussion by expanding on important ideas and events. For quick reference, a list of key facts concludes every chapter. Source notes, an annotated organizations list, bibliography, and index provide student researchers with additional tools for papers and class discussion.

The *In Controversy* series also challenges students to think critically about issues, to improve their problem-solving skills, and to sharpen their ability to form educated opinions. As President Barack Obama stated in a March 2009 speech, success in the twenty-first century will not be measurable merely by students' ability to "fill in a bubble on a test but whether they possess 21st century skills like problem-solving and critical thinking and entrepreneurship and creativity." Those who possess these skills will have a strong foundation for whatever lies ahead.

No one can know for certain what sort of world awaits today's students. What we can assume, however, is that those who are inquisitive about a wide range of issues; open-minded to divergent views; aware of bias and opinion; and able to reason, reflect, and reconsider will be best prepared for the future. As the international development organization Oxfam notes, "Today's young people will grow up to be the citizens of the future: but what that future holds for them is uncertain. We can be quite confident, however, that they will be faced with decisions about a wide range of issues on which people have differing, contradictory views. If they are to develop as global citizens all young people should have the opportunity to engage with these controversial issues."

In Controversy helps today's students better prepare for tomorrow. An understanding of the complex issues that drive our world and the ability to think critically about them are essential components of contributing, competing, and succeeding in the twenty-first century.

A Cautionary Tale

The story line of Kazuo Ishiguro's novel, *Never Let Me Go*, follows a group of school friends from childhood into adulthood. As children the characters attend a private boarding school in England called Hailsham, where art and physical activity are emphasized, but little else. The only adults at Hailsham are the teachers and the headmistress. As the novel progresses and the children grow older, however, the reader learns that these characters are clones of people living lives elsewhere. The sole purpose of these clones is to provide body parts for their aging counterparts. Depending on which organs or body parts the clones are needed for, they may only survive one, two, or three operations before they die.

An Ethical Debate

Though the book is science fiction, its theme—that science, in its pursuit of lifesaving and life-extending measures, can cross ethical lines—is at the very heart of the debate over embryonic stem cell (ESC) research. While blastocysts, the up-to-five-day-old embryos that are used in such research, are far from the fully developed people in Ishiguro's novel, opponents of stem cell research argue that a blastocyst is undeniably a potential human being, and the difference from it and a full-fledged human is simply a matter of time. To them, using such tissue is step one on the road to an ethical slippery slope in which society no longer views potential human beings as worthy of being called human. Deny that human blastocysts are human, many individuals claim, and people will grow to tolerate experiments on other human life, potentially even cloning humans for research or for replacement parts.

This idea, in fact, is not all that far-fetched, considering that when Dolly the sheep became the first mammal clone derived from an embryo created in a test tube in 1996, some very wealthy people paid to have a similar process used to clone a pet that had recently died. In fact, once Dolly's birth was announced, thousands of people, from homosexual couples to parents whose child had died, inquired whether they could use the technology to create a child clone. Today the technology for cloning humans does not exist, and animal cloning has a poor track record. When scientists have tried to clone animals, the failure rate remains 98 percent—embryos either never implant in the mother's uterus or they die off soon after implanting. Dolly, in fact, died only six years after her birth. Yet scientists continue to actively work on animal cloning.

Opponents of human ESC research maintain that all human life must be considered sacred from the first meeting of sperm and

A color-enhanced scanning electron micrograph reveals a human sperm (blue) fertilizing an egg. The meeting of sperm and egg lies at the heart of the debate over the ethics of human embryo experimentation.

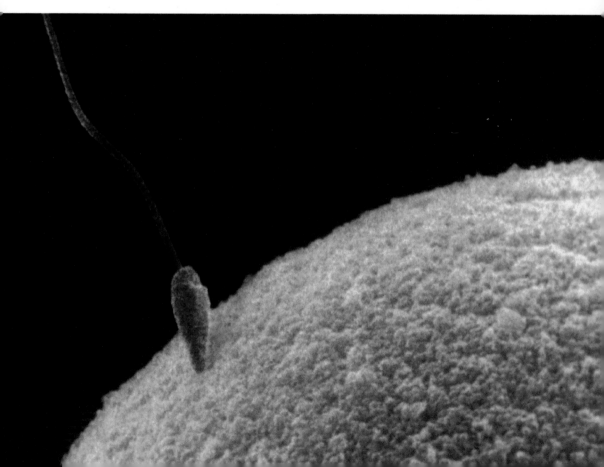

egg. They seek to distinguish human life as uniquely special and maintain that research that uses human tissue must be held up to a high moral standard. Many of these opponents are still champions of science, however, believing that scientists will find other ways to pursue their goals without the use of embryonic or fetal tissue. Indeed, the promise of adult stem cells seems to be proving this true.

New and Vital Treatments

Proponents of human ESC research argue that cloning has never been the objective. They contend that scientists instead are using such research to investigate human development and to cultivate cell lines to investigate new and vital treatments for conditions such as diabetes, Alzheimer's disease, Parkinson's disease, heart disease, spinal cord injury, and cancer. Denying scientists the ability to use these cells condemns thousands to continue without hope of a cure, advocates claim. Indeed, many scientists see arguments over cloning as a reflection of the ignorance of laypeople who do not understand the scientists' goals. And scientists are not alone in support of such research. People afflicted with diseases, their families, and their friends also rally behind ESC research, hoping that such cells can reverse these ailments.

While the probability of human cloning, then, seems far off, Ishiguro's novel echoes the concerns some people have over the ethics of stem cell research. When, in the novel, the headmistress is confronted by two clones who have fallen in love and want to know whether they can escape their fate, she tells them no. She explains, however, that while society no longer supports the experiment and clones are no longer used, their particular fate has been sealed. "You have to accept that sometimes that's how things happen in this world. People's opinions, their feelings, they go one way, then the other. It just so happens you grew up at a certain point in this process."[1] In today's scientific climate, opponents worry that just such compromises may be made in the zeal to help those who suffer from disease, while scientists argue that such conclusions are imaginary.

"Although often there is disagreement about matters of values, such disagreements are not evidence that values are simply subjective preferences, that they are groundless, or that agreement is not possible."[2]

— Philosophers Kristen K. Intemann and Inmaculada de Melo-Martin.

Ethics have always influenced the course of scientific progress, and debates over the value and costs of scientific pursuits have played out among scientists as well as within society at large. As philosophers Kristen K. Intemann and Inmaculada de Melo-Martin argue in the *FASEB Journal* of the Federation of American Societies for Experimental Biology, both scientists and society must contribute to the discussion: "Although often there is disagreement about matters of values, such disagreements are not evidence that values are simply subjective preferences, that they are groundless, or that agreement is not possible."[2] In the tension between scientific progress and ethical values, all of society may need to have a voice in the discussion to ensure that all viewpoints are heard.

What Are the Origins of the Human Embryo Experimentation Debate?

Research using human embryos is one of the most divisive ethical issues of the twenty-first century. From its onset human embryonic research has been hampered by moral questions. Some people regard any sort of experimentation on such cells as immoral because the cells are derived from embryos left over from in vitro fertilization (IVF) treatments. These people believe that such embryos should have the same moral status and rights as adult humans. Others have no such moral qualms, believing that because the cells hold such amazing potential to aid in new medical treatments, it is immoral not to pursue such research in the service of helping those suffering from debilitating diseases. These two sides have become intractable to the point that it is unlikely any sort of discussion about human embryonic research will yield agreement or compromise.

What Are Embryonic Stem Cells?

A human embryo is created by the union of a single male sperm cell and a female egg. After fertilization by the sperm cell, the egg begins to divide into more cells. These cells are called embryonic stem cells. All 210 types of human tissue eventually come from these cells. In the very early stages of embryo development, up to about five days after fertilization, ESCs are pluripotent, which means that they can be used to produce and replicate any type of adult cell in the body, such as bone, blood, muscle, or liver cells. Adults have a small number of stem cells, too, but most adult cells have already been assigned to a specific task in the body.

The cells from early embryos called blastocysts are much more versatile, however, and it is this versatility that makes the cells of great scientific interest. Researchers who work with ESCs believe that such cells have the potential to be inserted into the body to replace damaged or diseased cells to cure many human ailments. Diseases that researchers believe these cells could help are almost endless but include such major illnesses as heart disease, diabetes, and Parkinson's disease.

Scientists are also interested in why embryonic cells do what they do. For example, scientists hope to understand how these undifferentiated cells develop into specific tissues and organs. Thus, researchers look to stem cells for potentially providing valuable insights into disorders such as cancer or birth defects, which arise from abnormal differentiation and cell division. In addition, by cultivating stem cells, scientists hope they might discover that some cells have a predisposition to carry certain diseases. These cells could be grown in a lab and used to test new treatments. Finally, understanding the beginnings of cell life could yield a wealth of understanding about human health and growth. As University of Wisconsin science writer Terry Devitt says about such research, it is "the first window into the very earliest story of human development."[3]

Scientists have long known that some human cells were unusual, though they did not know exactly why. They knew, for example, that bone marrow was responsible for generating new blood. They even tried feeding bone marrow to patients afflicted with diseases of the blood, such as anemia and leukemia. Ingesting marrow did not work, but it was the first recognition that something was special about such human regeneration. In the 1950s scientists successfully experimented with mice to see if injecting them with bone marrow could cure them of radiation sickness. At the time, scientists did not know that bone marrow contained adult stem cells (ASCs); they thought instead that the marrow might contain a chemical that regenerated blood. These experiments eventually led to the discovery of ASCs in marrow during that decade. Scientists continued to research stem cells, with slow progress.

Embryonic-like stem cells were first discovered in human umbilical cord blood in 1978. As with ASCs, much of the research had its beginnings in animal models. In July 1981 Martin Evans and Matthew Kaufman from the Department of Genetics at the University of Cambridge culled the first in vitro stem cell lines from mice. Later that same year researcher Gail Martin at the University of California–San Francisco also demonstrated that embryonic-like stem cells could be developed from mouse embryos. It was Martin who coined the term *embryonic stem cells*.

Divisive Debate

Though research into embryonic-like stem cells had only just begun, embryonic research was quickly challenged in the courts. Antiabortion advocates led the way in publicizing and vilifying any research that used fetal tissue, arguing that such tissue was sacred. As early as 1974 Congress banned federally funded fetal tissue research until guidelines could be established. The same year, the federal government established the National Commission for the Protection of Human Subjects of Biomedical and Behavioral Research as part of the US Department of Health, Education, and Welfare. The commission's purpose is to establish policy regarding the protection of human subjects in general during medical experiments. Proponents of the commission, mostly religious conservatives, believed the guidelines that protect human subjects should also be fully extended to embryos.

Such legislation quieted most critics, and other scientific progress moved steadily on. The development of reproductive technologies, including IVF (that resulted in so-called test tube babies) in 1978, drew the attention of the federal government. These procedures generated ethical concerns because, again, they involve scientists purposely creating fertilized embryos for implantation.

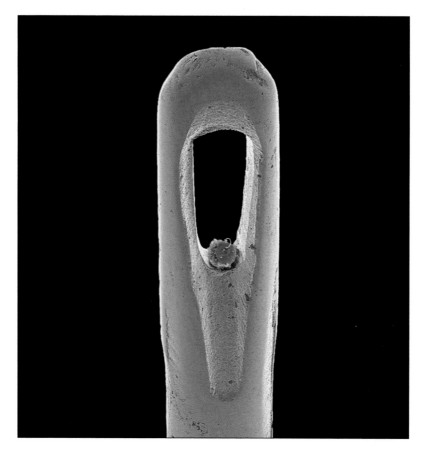

An embryonic stem cell (red) sits in the eye of a needle as seen through a colored scanning electron micrograph. ESCs are able to differentiate into any cell type—which is why they offer so much promise as a treatment for many serious illnesses.

Many such embryos are created in the process, but not all are used for implantation, so scientists were using the leftover embryos for research. This upset people who thought these embryos should be treated like human beings, albeit human beings who could not speak up about their fate. Thus, opponents argued, such embryos had a right not to be destroyed.

While the rights of embryos was certainly a major concern, another prominent fear was that scientists would go beyond using embryos for research and start to clone them. For years, scientists had been conducting research on cloning, or creating a living thing from another of its kind. As early as 1952, for example, researchers learned to clone small animal embryos such as those of frogs; many people saw this type of research as the beginning of a slippery slope toward cloning humans. The 1976 science-fiction novel and its subsequent movie *The Boys from Brazil,* in which neo-Nazis use Hitler's DNA to clone baby boys with the Nazi leader's genes, furthered such fears and suggested that the technology could easily lead to evil consequences. People worried that the virtual amorality of the pursuit of science would inevitably mean that scientists would not rest until they had successfully cloned humans. Though scientists argued that such fears were mere fantasies, people wanted the federal government to take more of a stand against such possibilities.

The two sides of the debate became more entrenched. Though a National Institutes of Health (NIH) panel voted in favor of government funding for embryo research in 1988, the government extended its ban on such research because of ethical concerns. Five years later, though, US Department of Health and Human Services secretary Donna Shalala lifted the moratorium on stem cell research following an executive order by President Bill Clinton, and Congress voted to override the moratorium on government funding of ESC research. Thousands of people wrote letters urging Clinton to reverse his decision, which he did the following year.

> "The birth of Dolly would raise a troubling issue: the prospect of human cloning. . . . This possibility would engender a wide range of questions about the purposes, applications, and ethics of modern biological research."[5]
>
> — Harold Varmus, former director of the NIH.

By 1996 Congress had banned federal funding for embryonic research that destroyed the embryo with the so-called Dickey-Wicker Amendment, which prohibited the use of federal money for "the creation of a human embryo or embryos for research purposes; or research in which a human embryo or embryos are destroyed, discarded, or knowingly subjected to risk of injury or death greater than that allowed for research on fetuses in utero [in the uterus]."[4] The Dickey-Wicker Amendment continues to guide human stem cell research today.

In 1996 the birth of the first cloned mammal, Dolly the sheep, relit the fire over stem cells and their role in cloning. As Harold Varmus, former director of the NIH, said: "For the general public . . . the birth of Dolly would raise a troubling issue: the prospect of human cloning. . . . This possibility would engender a wide range of questions about the purposes, applications, and ethics of modern biological research."[5] For opponents, the creation of Dolly

Somatic Cell Nuclear Transfer

Many scientists seeking medical breakthroughs support somatic cell nuclear transfer, a procedure that involves transferring a cell nucleus into a donated egg to create an embryo from which stem cells can be culled. Like so many aspects of the stem cell debate, somatic cell nuclear transfer, also called therapeutic cloning, is fraught with controversy. Among supporters of this technology is Thomas Okarma, president of Geron Corporation, who issued the following statement on June 20, 2001, before the US House Subcommittee on Health:

> Our nation is on the cusp of reaping the long dreamed-of rewards from our significant investment in biomedical research. The U.S. biotech industry is the envy of much of the world, especially our ability to turn basic research at NIH and universities into applied research at biotech companies and, in turn, into new therapies and cures for individual patients. Using somatic cell nuclear transfer and other cloning technologies, biotech researchers will continue to learn about cell differentiation, re-programming and other areas of cell and molecular biology. Armed with this information, they can eventually crack the codes of diseases and conditions that have plagued us for hundreds of years, indeed, for millennia.

Thomas Okarma, testimony before the Subcommittee on Health, House Judiciary Committee, June 20, 2001. www.appropriations.senate.gov.

was their biggest nightmare realized. Though banned from cloning humans, scientists had succeeded in cloning animals, which critics believed was just as bad. Dolly only lived six years, however, when most sheep live eleven or twelve years. This also raised fears.

Many critics took the example of Dolly to bolster their argument that scientists would not stop to think of the ethical issues cloning raised; they would merely do whatever the federal government allowed them to do. Opponents argued that without strict government regulation, scientists would run amok.

A New Era of Political Controversy

The debate about embryonic research intensified in 1998, when a group of biologists at the University of Wisconsin–Madison, led by James Thomson, first isolated and cultured human ESCs, establishing five stem cell lines. The group proved that these cell lines could be proliferated in cell cultures and then developed into many different types of cells. With this discovery—that ESCs had the unique ability to specialize into different body tissues—the issue of regulation became even more controversial. Scientists argued that stem cell research had tremendous potential in disease treatment, and many wanted Congress to rethink the stem cell ban on the grounds that it hindered potentially lifesaving research. At the same time, people objected to the fact that the process Thomson used in his experiments destroyed the embryos and therefore violated the sanctity of life.

Despite questions regarding the fate of the embryos, research continued, and other discoveries soon followed. Most of this research showed that scientists were gaining knowledge in how stem cells became differentiated and proliferated. In the same year that Thomson isolated stem cells, John Gearhart from Johns Hopkins University developed pluripotent stem cell lines from fetal gonad tissue, proving that certain specific fetal cells could be manipulated to become independent pluripotent cells. In 1999 and 2000 still other researchers discovered that they could manipulate certain types of adult mouse tissue to produce different cell types. These discoveries were crucial to the burgeoning field of stem cell research. Both studies proved that human stem cells could be sustained in culture and replicated through generations without losing their versatility.

Both researchers followed the strict guidelines governing stem cell research. Both did their research using private funding. Thomson obtained embryos from a fertility clinic that was going to dispose of them. Gearhart used fetal cells that had been donated to science, and he obtained proper permission. Both hoped to eliminate any doubt that they were acting legally and ethically. Yet opponents still objected.

The Moral Debate Spawns New Regulations

Despite these exciting findings, many objections to stem cell research focused on the fact that stem cell therapies remained unproven. Scientists had yet to develop concrete, successful stem cell treatments for disease using stem cells, and many challenges and risks had to be overcome before such research could be considered valid science. Because it remained theoretical, opponents believed that researchers had an even larger obligation to err in favor of the sanctity of life and refuse to experiment on potential human beings. These critics believed that scientists were sacrificing human lives for the unproven possibility of saving other lives. As before, the fact that taking stem cells from embryos results in the destruction of the embryos remained at the center of the debate.

With these concerns in mind, the NIH took action soon after Thomson first isolated human ESCs in 1998. In 2000 the agency developed guidelines for funding human ESC research. The NIH still believed such research was necessary and could be moral within certain parameters. In a press release about their guidelines for using human pluripotent stem cells in research, the NIH stated:

"[ESC] research promises new treatments and possible cures for many debilitating diseases and injuries, including Parkinson's disease, diabetes, heart disease, multiple sclerosis, burns and spinal cord injuries."[6]

— National Institutes of Health, an agency of the US Department of Health and Human Services.

> Such research promises new treatments and possible cures for many debilitating diseases and injuries, including Parkinson's disease, diabetes, heart disease, multiple sclerosis, burns and spinal cord injuries. The NIH believes the potential medical benefits of human pluripotent stem cell technology are compelling and worthy of pursuit in accordance with appropriate ethical standards.[6]

The NIH guidelines stipulated that federal funds could be applied to research on stem cell lines derived from embryos created with private funds and left over from fertility clinics. When George W. Bush won the presidential election later that same year, he narrowed the parameters of what research would be considered eligible for federal funds, including requiring researchers to prove that the embryos they used were obtained with the informed consent of the parent.

Federal approval of stem cell research has been an important step in legitimizing stem cell research. For one, obtaining the number of embryos required to further stem cell lines requires that the government give the approval for a consistent procurement system. Secondly, because experimental research offers no concrete product or treatment to attract a lot of private monies and investors, federal funding ensures that universities, for example, can have the funds to continue the research. Such venues need federal funding to pay for equipment, fund graduate students to help with the research, and other crucial expenses. When the federal government withdraws funds from scientific research, in many cases it is virtually impossible for publicly funded institutions to continue to move ahead, or it makes progress extremely slow.

Regulation in the Bush Era

The NIH decision was a significant aspect of George W. Bush's presidency. Bush was a strong supporter of the right-to-life movement. He believed that life should be vigorously protected, even in its earliest stages. On August 9, 2001, Bush announced his decision to curtail government funding for the ESC lines not already in existence as of that year but not to restrict funding of ASC research, which does not require the destruction of human embryos. Bush stated, "I . . . believe human life is a sacred gift from our Creator. I worry about a culture that devalues life, and believe as your President I have an important obligation to foster and encourage respect for life in America and throughout the world."[7] Although

Bush did not actually ban ESC research—he merely stated that no federal funds would be available to support new research that would foster the future destruction of embryos—many researchers felt that these prohibitions limited scientific inquiry, particularly as some of the stem cell lines in existence had not been tested long enough and were of dubious quality.

Scientists kept trying to modify the Bush edict by asking for further modifications. Because most Americans at the time supported stem cell research (and continue to do so today), petitions encouraged Congress to ease restrictions. Many legislators were swayed by the public outcry. In 2005 Congress approved the Stem Cell Research Enhancement Act, a bill that would permit federal funding of stem cell research on human embryos that were left over from in vitro fertilization. The following year, however, Bush vetoed this legislation, justifying his decision by reiterating his moral concerns.

Bush had been elected in part by the powerful antiabortion lobby, and he believed he represented that lobby. Some criticized the president for simply pandering to the powerful group. As Graeme Laurie of Edinburgh University commented on Bush's decision:

> The stated reason for President Bush's objection to embryonic stem cell research is that "murder is wrong"; why then does he not intervene to regulate or ban [embryonic] stem cell research carried out with private funds and which is happening across the US? . . . It is a strange morality indeed that pins the moral status and life of the embryo on the question of who is paying for the research.[8]

Despite these arguments, stem cell research continued to progress, with countless research studies showing that ESCs have the potential to be useful in treating disease. Since scientists have only been able to experiment on ESCs since 1998, when Thomson first demonstrated how to isolate and grow these specialized cells, the research is still in its infancy, with many unknowns.

For example, it remains unclear how transplanted stem cells will affect humans. Some of the research appears to show that treatments are not always beneficial. When mice with Parkinson's

A Slippery Slope

The National Right to Life Committee (NRLC) is one of the nation's most prominent pro-life groups. When Barack Obama signed an executive order on March 31, 2009, to allow federal funding of research that would require the destruction of human embryos, the NRLC issued a scathing response the same day. The NRLC condemned Obama's order on the grounds that advances in research using nonembryonic sources rendered ESC research unnecessary. The group also voiced concern that this move would create a slippery slope that would encourage the widespread killing of embryonic life. As Douglas Johnson, a spokesperson for the group, said:

> It is a sad day when the federal government will fund research that exploits living members of the human species as raw material for research. Obama's order also places our society on a very steep, very slippery slope. Many researchers will not be satisfied to use only so-called surplus embryos. Many researchers are already demanding federal support for research in which human embryos would be created for the specific purpose of research, through human cloning and other methods, and there was nothing in the President's remark today to limit NIH to the use of so-called surplus embryos created in IVF clinics.

National Right to Life, "Obama Order Opens Door to Widespread Killing of Embryonic Humans in Government-Funded Research," March 9, 2009. www.nrlc.org.

disease were injected with stem cells, for example, they developed brain tumors. Another worry that has emerged is that transplanted ESCs could be attacked by a patient's own immune system. Some of these concerns might be mitigated as new studies begin to address these shortcomings. One of the options for preventing rejection, for example, focuses on creating ESCs through therapeutic cloning, which renders stem cells that are genetically identical to the patient's cells and thereby minimizes the risk of rejection.

A Call for Alternate Sources

With debate raging during the Bush presidency about the ethics of using ESCs, other research started to focus on ASCs. ASCs are not always pluripotent, but many can differentiate into some of the specialized cell types of major tissues or organs and therefore have potential restorative powers. At a 2004 Senate hearing on ASC research, two women who had been paralyzed in automobile accidents were able to walk into the hearing room. The two had been treated in Portugal with a procedure pioneered by Dr. Carlos Lima. In this groundbreaking surgery, doctors transplanted stem cells derived from the women's own olfactory tissue into the spinal cord at the injury site. There they formed new nerve cells, allowing the women to walk again. While the demonstration was dramatic, many remain unconvinced. Critics pointed out that spontaneous recovery in spinal cord injuries sometimes occurs without treatment of any kind. In response to these and other accounts, Bush urged support for research on ASCs and other nonembryonic sources of pluripotent cells.

A novel discovery in 2007 also seemed to staunch the moral debate. Working independently of one another, Shinya Yamanaka of Kyoto University in Japan and James Thomson of the University of Wisconsin–Madison in the United States discovered a technique to inject genetic material into skin cells by way of a virus and make the cells behave like ESCs. Researchers were able to coax these special skin cells to take on the role of nerve cells and living heart cells.

These cells, called induced pluripotent stem cells, hold great promise because they would eliminate the need to harvest pluripotent stem cells from human embryos, removing the ethical hurdles to further research. Researchers continue to perfect these techniques so that someday these cells can become widely available. In 2009, for example, researchers in Edinburgh and Toronto

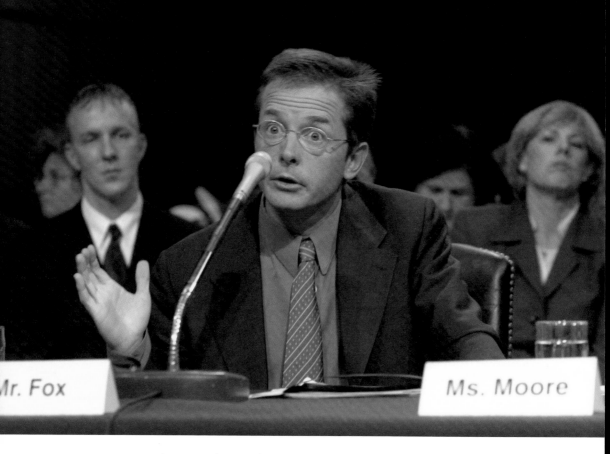

Mr. Fox

Ms. Moore

Actor Michael J. Fox testifies before a Senate subcommittee about the importance of stem cell research in efforts to cure debilitating diseases. Fox, who has Parkinson's disease (a nervous system disorder that worsens over time), supports increased federal funding for this research.

discovered a method that can induce pluripotent cells that does not require the use of a virus, which makes it far safer for practical use. As research continues, future doctors may be able to create new heart, brain, or spinal cord cells that originate from a patient's own skin cells.

First Human Trials

Proponents of stem cell research say that these practical results are what are required to end the controversy; they argue that if scientists can achieve concrete results, then more people would see the clear benefits. Such stakeholders in the debate could speak for themselves on the value of their treatment. Actor Michael J. Fox, who contracted Parkinson's disease, has become an advocate for stem cell research and a visible spokesperson for the cause. Founder of the Michael J. Fox Foundation for Parkinson's Research, Fox is well liked and personable. The actor has testified before Congress and regularly lobbies for increased funding of stem cell research, often after not taking his medications in order to show the devastating effects of the disease. Fox states: "I can't think of a greater affirmation of the culture of life than to advance the fight against disease by increasing federal funding for biomedical research."[9]

Largely in response to such eloquent pleas from patients and supporters, the US Food and Drug Administration (FDA) approved clinical trials in January 2009 for transplanting a certain type of brain and spinal cord cell (derived from ESCs) into individuals who had recently suffered spinal cord injury. In October 2010 researchers from Geron Corporation in Menlo Park, California, administered these ESCs to the first human patient. Researchers hoped that the new cells would replicate within the body and restore some level of spinal cord function. As Geron's president, Thomas Okarma, said, "Embryonic stem cells are really nature's own way of making more of ourselves. We are simply harnessing the biology of normal human development in our attempts to achieve permanent cures to chronic disease and injury."[10]

Before any definitive results could be gleaned, however, Geron announced that it was halting stem cell research to pursue cancer research, largely for financial reasons. Patients with spinal cord injuries and others felt a huge letdown, interpreting Geron's move as a step backward for research. As Robert Lanza, chief scientific officer of Advanced Cell Technology, commented: "To have the first group out the door throw their hat in doesn't sound good. . . . We need a big success. Someone has to show that it really works. Until that happens, a lot of people will be skeptical."[11]

Such a breakthrough may be forthcoming since other studies using human subjects are under way. A team of researchers from the University of California–Los Angeles and Advanced Cell Technology are conducting a series of clinical trials that will assess the safety of using stem cell therapy to treat patients with macular degeneration, the leading cause of blindness in the United States. Preliminary reports hint that the treatment is safe and effective, although it is far too early for any definitive conclusions to be drawn.

"I can't think of a greater affirmation of the culture of life than to advance the fight against disease by increasing federal funding for biomedical research."[9]

— Actor and ESC research supporter Michael J. Fox.

In March 2009 newly elected president Barack Obama promised to modify the Bush administration's restrictions on stem cell research. When he signed an executive order titled Removing Barriers to Responsible Scientific Research Involving Human Stem Cells, Obama stated, "Today, with the Executive Order I am about to sign . . . we will lift the ban on federal funding for promising embryonic stem cell research. We will vigorously support scientists who pursue this research. And we will aim for America to lead the world in the discoveries it one day may yield."[12] Whether Obama's softened stance will lead to more public acceptance is unknown. For now, it appears too early to determine whether science will be able to harness the power of stem cells to treat disease. As the field continues to progress, debate among scientists, the public, government officials, and religious groups will continue to guide policy on research and treatment procedures.

Facts

- The late actor Christopher Reeve used his celebrity to further ESC research after he suffered a severe spinal cord injury that left him paralyzed. He died in 2004.

- In 2011, the largest study to date on stem cell therapy used a patient's own bone marrow stem cells to repair damaged heart tissue and may pave the way for future treatments for heart disease.

- In 2012 researchers reported in the *Journal of the American Medical Association* that ASCs in bone marrow may replace powerful antirejection drugs in transplant recipients.

- Federal funding for ESC research nearly doubled between 2008 and 2010 (from $88.1 million to $165.2 million), largely due to Barack Obama's changes in policy governing this type of research.

- An estimated $128 million will be supplied by the NIH to fund ESC research in 2012.

- In 2010 the NIH provided $415 million for nonembryonic human stem cell research.

- In 2001 scientists from Advanced Cell Technology announced the cloning of the first human embryos for therapeutic research.

CHAPTER TWO

Is Human Embryo Experimentation Moral?

At the heart of the debate over the morality of stem cell research lies the antiabortion debate. Stem cell research destroys human embryos, and those who are opposed to abortion, including many religious groups, believe it is morally wrong to destroy any human life, including the potential life of an embryo. Others argue that it is morally wrong to allow many who suffer from diseases such as diabetes, spinal cord injury, Parkinson's, and Alzheimer's to be denied the hope for a cure that the potential of such research could yield.

Though stem cell research uses embryos that have already been created and are either voluntarily donated or, because they are about to be destroyed, donated to science, abortion foes still see their use as wrong. As D.C. Wertz at the University of Massachusetts Medical School writes: "The US has a politically active anti-abortion movement that came to life after [the 1973 US Supreme Court case] *Roe v Wade* legalized elective abortion. Stem cell research is irretrievably linked with the abortion debate and probably always will be."[13]

Those who support stem cell research do not argue that human embryos should be used without any ethical boundaries. Many believe that they do treat human tissue with respect and never forget that they are dealing with a sensitive issue. A pioneer in stem cell research, James Thomson, says, "If human embryonic stem cell research does not make you at least a little bit uncomfortable, you have not thought about it enough. . . . I thought long and hard about whether I would do it."[14]

Should an Embryo Be Considered a Person with Full Human Rights?

Stem cells come from human embryos that are four or five days old. At this early stage of development, they consist of about one hundred to two hundred cells, that have not begun to differentiate into the cells that will form the brain, heart, and other parts of a person. To those who believe that human life begins at conception, this small cluster of embryonic cells represents a sacred, distinct, human life. Destroying the embryo to yield stem cells is tantamount to murder.

Those who oppose stem cell research offer several arguments in their defense. While many of these detractors are religious, not all of the arguments are. One argument is that science is amoral and thus cannot be in charge of nor draw up guidelines that involve moral issues. Because scientists must pursue a secular goal, the advancement of scientific possibilities, they must be reined in when it comes to sensitive moral issues such as using human embryos in research. Like many religions that consider the embryo a person with full rights, the Catholic Church squarely put forth its views after George W. Bush's statement outlining the parameters of federal funding for ESC research in 2001. As Pope John Paul II said: "Experience is already showing how a tragic coarsening of consciences accompanies the assault on innocent human life in the womb, leading to accommodation and acquiescence in the face of other related evils such as euthanasia, infanticide and, most recently, proposals for the creation for research purposes of human embryos, destined to be destroyed in the process."[15]

Bishop Joseph A. Fiorenza agrees that stem cell research is

"If human embryonic stem cell research does not make you at least a little bit uncomfortable, you have not thought about it enough."[14]

— Stem cell pioneer James Thomson.

a step toward favoring a scientific view over its moral problems. "The federal government, for the first time in history, will support research that relies on the destruction of some defenseless human beings for the possible benefit to others. However such a decision is hedged about with qualification, it allows our nation's research enterprise to cultivate a disrespect for human life."[16]

Another piece to the anti–stem cell argument is biological. Because the human embryo is biologically pre-destined to become a human life, some people argue that there should be the same safeguards and rights for an embryo as for any human subjects in experiments. There is no time when an embryo starts to be human, these people argue. It is human from conception. Robert P. George and Christopher Tollefsen write in their book, *Embryo: A Defense of Human Life*:

A human embryo is a whole living member of the species Homo sapiens in the earliest stage of his or her development. Unless severely damaged, or denied or deprived of a suitable environment, a human being in the embryonic stage will, by directing its own integral organic functioning, develop himself or herself to the next more mature developmental stage, i.e., the fetal stage.[17]

Those who make this argument are particularly annoyed by those who argue that the embryo is only a potential human life. For example, Scott Klusendorf, president of the pro-life Life Training Institute, says, "Embryos don't come from stem cells; they are living human beings that have stem cells. And extracting these cells is lethal for the tiny human subject."[18]

Opponents of stem cell research take the biological argument further. Because a human embryo has to be considered a human from conception, it must be endowed with certain human rights, including the primary right not to be destroyed. Unlike adults, embryos are inducted into research without their consent. This makes such research immoral on its face, say many opponents, including Gilbert Meilaender, a professor of Christian ethics at

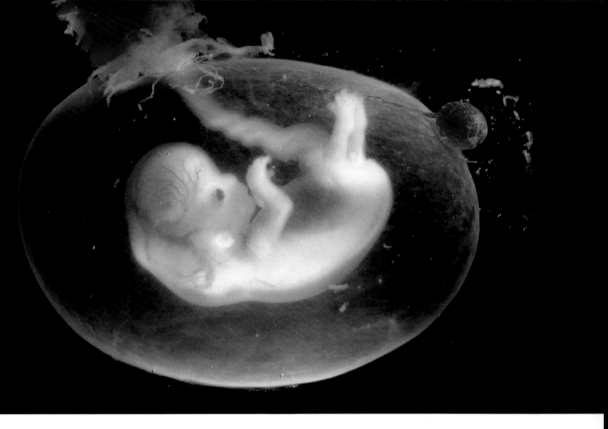

Valparaiso University in Indiana. He contends, "Using embryos that can't consent to research is equivalent to forcibly drafting any other human being to be an experimental research subject."[19] Meilaender and others liken embryos to other vulnerable members of society, such as children or people with mental or physical disabilities. For the same reasons that a moral society does not use its most vulnerable members to achieve its own ends—including the possibilities of ending their lives because they are a burden to society or experimenting on them because they are less valuable than healthy individuals—society must also protect human embryos, which are equally vulnerable.

Thus, self-awareness should not determine whether humans have value, opponents maintain; otherwise, newborns, for example, would not qualify for the full range of human rights. George and Tollefsen argue that it is this slippery slope that needs to be kept in mind when discussing society's responsibility for all of its members. This responsibility is not lessened by the promise of great benefits to some. They write:

At ten weeks of development, the embryo clearly shows human characteristics. Embryonic stem cell research involves embryos from a much earlier stage of development. This does not matter to critics, who believe the destruction of any embryo is the same as taking a human life.

Amidst the promises of boundless health benefits from this research, it can become tempting to lose sight of all that is really at stake. But consider the following analogy. Suppose that a movement arose to obtain transplantable organs by killing mentally retarded infants. Would the controversy that would inevitably erupt over this be best characterized as a debate about organ transplantation? Would anyone accept as a legitimate description the phrase therapeutic organ harvesting? Surely not: the dispute would best be characterized—and in any decent society it would be characterized—as a debate about the ethics of killing retarded children in order to obtain their organs.[20]

Pro-Research Views

Stem cell advocates do not deny that embryos are human; they make distinctions to argue that at the time when such embryos are the most valuable to research—one to five days after conception—it is difficult to say that such a cluster of cells is equal to a complete human being. Supporters argue that these tiny blastocysts with no human features whatsoever cannot merit the same human rights of people already living. Arthur Caplan, a professor of medical ethics at the University of Pennsylvania, argues, "An embryo in a dish is more like a set of instructions or blueprint for a house. It can't build the house. For the cells to develop into a human being requires an interactive process in the uterus between the embryo and the mother."[21] These embryos are not created in nature, after all, and they have no way of sustaining themselves outside of a researcher keeping them alive. Such an artificial process proves that embryos are not the equivalent of humans that develop in a woman's uterus, these advocates argue. "If you were to leave that fertilized blastocyst in the petri dish and provide it with nutrients and go away for a trip to the beach, you won't come back and find your son or daughter in the petri dish. . . . It will reach a stage where it will simply die,"[22] contends Gary Pettett, a neonatologist at the Center for Practical Bioethics in Kansas City, Missouri.

Fourteen Days: An Important Marker for Life

Because of these issues, many people believe it is important to define the moment that life begins. Many biologists view fourteen days as the marker for when life begins, since that is when an embryo becomes a distinct, single individual. According to Ronald A. Lindsey, president of the Center for Inquiry, which promotes the advancement of science:

> *The early embryo is not an individual.* Until about 14 days after conception, the embryo can divide into two or more parts. Under the right conditions, each of those parts can develop into a separate fetus. This is the phenomenon known as "twinning." Twinning shows that adult human beings are not identical with a previously existing zygote [the cell that is formed after an egg is fertilized] or embryo. If that were true, then each pair of twins would be identical with the same embryo. This is a logically incoherent position. If A and B are separate individuals, they cannot both be identical with a previously existent entity, C. As the early embryo is not an individual, it cannot be the moral equivalent of an adult human. To claim that someone is harmed, there must be "someone" there. We do not and should not grant moral rights to mere groupings of cells.[23]

"We do not and should not grant moral rights to mere groupings of cells."[23]

— Ronald A. Lindsey, president of the Center for Inquiry, an organization that promotes the advancement of science.

The fourteenth day of gestation is an important landmark for other reasons, as well. Not only do the cells develop enough that the possibility of twinning disappears, but other important characteristics, such as the ability to sense, begin, albeit at a very primitive state. Jane Maienschein, the director of the Center for Biology and Society at Arizona State University, asserts:

> For many biologists, biologically meaningful life begins only after the biologically significant stage called "gastrulation" [the early stage when an embryo is dramatically restructured by cell migration]. . . . Soon after gastrulation comes development of the "primitive streak." This stage

occurs by the fourteenth day, and it is marked by the appearance of differentiated cells that apparently have some capacity to experience sensation. This capacity to feel offers a point of difference that many believe is the meaningful beginning of a real life.[24]

Beyond the argument that blastocysts do not constitute biologically significant life is the fact that every one of the embryos used in stem cell research is already artificially created. They were

Creating Embryos for Research

Leon Kass is the author of *The Ethics of Human Cloning*. Kass believes that the creation of embryos via therapeutic cloning—with the intent of destroying them for the alleged benefit of others—displays a profound disrespect for human life. Kass writes:

> "The prospect of creating new human life solely to be exploited in this way has been condemned on moral grounds by many people . . . as displaying a profound disrespect for life. Even those who are willing to scavenge so-called "spare embryos"— those products of in vitro fertilization made in excess of people's reproductive needs, and otherwise likely to be discarded—draw back from creating human embryos explicitly and solely for research purposes. They reject outright what they regard as the exploitation and the instrumentalization of nascent human life. In addition, others who are agnostic about the moral status of the embryo see the wisdom of not . . . offending the sensibilities of their fellow citizens who are opposed to such practices."

Leon Kass, "Preventing a Brave New World," *New Republic Online*, June 21, 2001. www.tnr.com.

created in a petri dish to serve human ends—that is, to help an infertile couple become pregnant. Without this artificial scientific intervention, such embryos would not exist at all. As University of Albany ethics expert Bonnie Steinbock argues, this distinction alone makes such cells less than human. She claims that in IVF procedures, "embryos are created for our purposes. If it is wrong to create embryos that will be destroyed, this applies not merely to embryos created for research, but also to embryos created for reproduction. If one takes seriously the notion of protecting the lives of extracorporeal [outside the body] embryos, then one ought not to create any surplus embryos."[25]

In IVF, Steinbock claims, embryos are created to aid in a significant and important end: reproduction. Just like reproduction, scientific advancement should also be seen as an important, if not noble, goal. As she states: "Medical research that has the potential to prolong and improve people's lives is at least as valuable as enabling infertile people to become parents."[26]

Steinbock's assertion is perhaps the most significant argument that stem cell advocates make: that such research has the potential to cure disease. These advocates wonder how society can turn its back on such research that might benefit the living for such almost purely philosophical arguments about when life begins. For example, geneticists Stanley Fields and Mark Johnston believe that stem cells can one day cure diabetes. They further believe that embryos are not people and therefore do not have rights that trump those of people suffering debilitating diseases that could be alleviated by stem cell therapies. In their book, *Genetic Twists of Fate*, the authors explain their view:

> Scientists have a duty to prevent or alleviate human suffering, with the utmost importance placed on saving the lives of people already among us. An embryo consisting of one hundred to two hundred cells—about the size of the period at the end of this sentence—has no brain or central nervous system and no other organs associated with a person. This lack of sentience [awareness] is an argument that this tiny embryo should not have the same status and

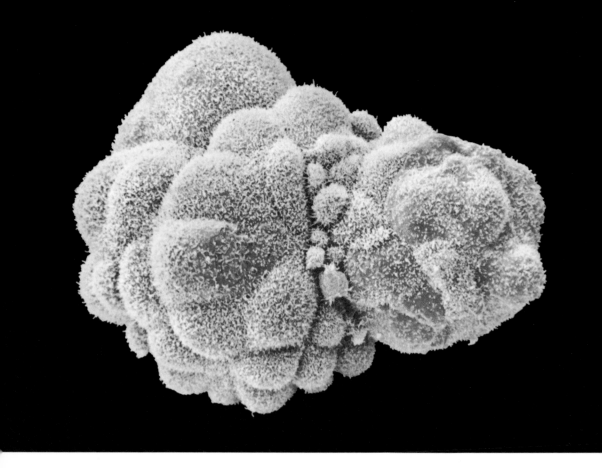

Six days after fertilization a human embryo, or blastocyst, is basically a collection of cells—visible only through a colored scanning electron micrograph. The blastocyst begins to develop only after it is implanted on the uterine wall.

rights as a living person. Of course, the embryo must be given serious respect, and strict controls must be in place to limit its use to research that can benefit humanity. But we should not abandon the tremendous potential of embryonic stem cells for curing disease.[27]

Surplus Embryos

Advocates argue also that most of the embryos used to cull stem cells are left over from fertility clinics and are destined to be destroyed or remain frozen indefinitely. In fact, fertility doctors deliberately create far more embryos than are needed. In this way they are able to select the embryos that are the healthiest and the most likely to implant and develop into a full-term fetus. This process, however, results in the destruction of many embryos—many more, in fact, than are destroyed in stem cell research. Although difficult to quantify precisely, some estimate that up to six hundred thousand surplus embryos remain frozen at fertility clinics across the country, and around eight thousand to ten thousand of these are discarded each year. Such wanton destruction leads many in the pro-research camp to argue that their opponents are hypocritical. Michael Kinsley, who supports ESC research, observes, "If embryos are human beings with full human rights, fertility clinics are death camps—with a side order of cold-blooded eugenics. No one who truly believes in the humanity of embryos could possibly think otherwise."[28]

On the other hand, if stem cell research can be a moral choice, then would it not be better for such embryos to be used to promote life? As Louis Guenin of the International Society for Stem Cell Research argues in his book, *The Morality of Embryo Use*: "If there's even a chance that the embryos that are currently being discarded are used in some way that can benefit people, that's a good ethical choice."[29]

If anything, opponents argue, these frozen embryos should be adopted rather than discarded or used for research. According to the Embryo Adoption Awareness Center, more than three thousand babies have been born through these egg adoption programs since the first one was established in 1997. Embryo adoptions continue to increase—they were up 27 percent from 2010 to 2011. This very process is significant to opponents, including ethicist Amy Coxon. She writes, "The fact that 'excess' frozen embryos can be adopted and allowed to develop into fully functioning members of the human race also indicates that these embryos are not just potential human beings. In fact, these embryos truly are the smallest and most vulnerable people in our society, and they should be given the same respect as any other member of society."[30]

"If there's even a chance that the embryos that are currently being discarded are used in some way that can benefit people, that's a good ethical choice."[29]

— Louis Guenin, author of *The Morality of Embryo Use*.

Do Stem Cell Lines and ASCs Negate the Need?

Bush attempted a compromise between the two opposing camps when he limited ESC research to cell lines that had already been created before 2001. To many proponents, using stem cell lines such as these, which do not involve the future destruction of any embryos, trumps the opposition's arguments.

Yet the very nature of science, especially new science, means that many stem cell lines developed before 2001 are no longer very useful to scientists today, who know so much more about keeping such lines healthy and versatile. Fields and Johnston describe the hurdles scientists face when using these existing stem cell lines:

> Almost all the existing [stem cell lines] are flawed. Many seem to have limited potential, being able to give rise to only certain types of cells. Worse, many of the stem-cell lines that exist today are contaminated, precluding their use in humans. They were grown on a layer of mouse cells, to provide factors necessary for stem cell growth. . . . Biologists have learned much about the care and handling of embryonic stem cells in the last several years, promising healthier, more versatile, and more consistent stem-cell lines in the future.[31]

"Embryos truly are the smallest and most vulnerable people in our society, and they should be given the same respect as any other member of society."[30]

— Ethicist Amy Coxon, member of the Center for Bioethics and Human Dignity.

The restrictions that these lines have placed on scientists, in fact, have led many to attempt to circumvent their use. Some scientists have been devoting research time to reprogramming adult cells to return to an earlier, unspecialized state. This new research, scientists hope, will one day negate the need for human ESCs. As Senators Bob Smith, Sam Brownback, and Tim Hutchinson write: "It is becoming more and more difficult to defend medical research which uses tissue derived from abortions or from the destruction of human embryos, when breakthroughs using alternative sources of tissue are being made in the medical research community."[32] The controversy, however, is not likely to end soon, as many scientists believe that the study of ESCs will continue to remain crucial. These noncontroversial approaches will require years of development before they are a viable alternative, if indeed ever. For one thing, ASCs are extremely difficult to find in the body. In addition, they must be greatly manipulated to be of use. After ASCs are removed, they must be maintained and grown in

Spontaneous Abortion and the Stem Cell Debate

Ronald A. Lindsey, president of the Center for Inquiry, an organization that promotes the advancement of science, explains why be believes that arguments against ESC research are illogical:

> The claim that the embryo is the moral equivalent of a human person is implicitly rejected by *everyone*. One important fact about embryonic development that is often overlooked is that between two-thirds and four-fifths of all embryos that are generated through standard sexual reproduction are spontaneously aborted. If embryos have the same status as human persons, this is a horrible tragedy and public health crisis that requires immediate and sustained attention. Not only should we abandon stem cell research, but we should reallocate the vast majority of our research dollars from projects such as cancer research into programs to help prevent this staggering loss of human life. Interestingly, none of the opponents of embryonic stem cell research have called for research programs that might increase the odds of embryo survival. Their failure to address this issue is puzzling if the embryo deserves the same moral respect as human persons.

Ronald A. Lindsey, "Adult Reasoning About Embryos," Center for Inquiry, August 27, 2010. www.centerforinquiriy.net.

tissue culture for long periods of time. Because it takes a long time, changes can occur in the cells that render them useless.

Yet other scientists are not willing to give up on ASCs, and they believe the potential of ASCs is just as great as that of ESCs.

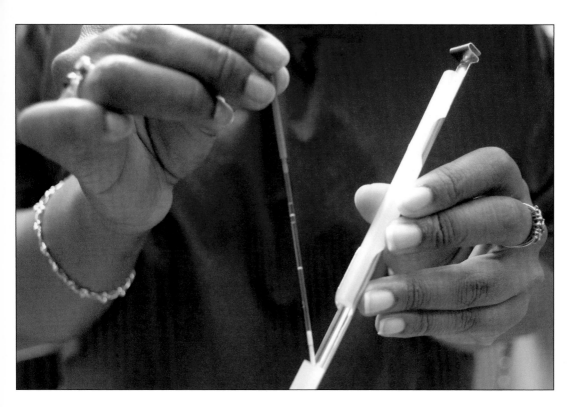

Frozen embryos are stored in long white tubes such as this one at a California fertility clinic. Thousands of surplus embryos from fertility clinics are either destroyed or frozen indefinitely.

According to Robert Lanza of Advanced Cell Technology, "It's not practical to use right now, but it might be in a few years. This is truly the Holy Grail—to be able to take a few cells from a patient—say a cheek swab or few skin cells—and turn them into stem cells in the laboratory."[33]

In fact, some experiments with skin cells are showing such promise, argues Theresa Deisher, that they are actually producing results, while ESC research has no record of healing. Deisher and others assert that scientists should give up the pursuit of the morally difficult ESC research and simply begin to devote themselves wholeheartedly to ASCs.

Determining Public Policy

It is clear that no matter what research scientists ultimately pursue, guidelines and oversight will remain important as the many ethical quandaries are sorted out in the years ahead. Do No Harm: The Coalition of Americans for Research Ethics is one organization that promotes ethical scientific research and health care. As the coalition's communication's director Gene Tarne and his colleague David Prentice write:

> In an open society, determining public policy on science requires hearing from many voices, voices from outside the scientific community such as ethicists, religious leaders, economists, philosophers, and others, in addition to members of the scientific community. The perspectives they bring should not and must not be dismissed as ideological, sectarian, or narrow-minded. Just as war is too important to leave to the generals, setting public policy on science is too important to leave to the scientists.[34]

Many organizations continue to monitor the stem cell field, including technological advances and the development of new procedures that may change the nature of the debate. The National Academies, a collection of private, nonprofit public policy advice centers, has published guidelines, for example, that require institutional review boards and oversight committees to ensure that research is carried out in an ethical way. For now, the debate about the moral status of the human embryo continues, for, as Louis Guenin puts it, "There is no test for whether an embryo is a person. Instead we are left to our own devices, to our own moral reasoning."[35]

> "There is no test for whether an embryo is a person. Instead we are left to our own devices, to our own moral reasoning."[35]
>
> — Louis Guenin, author of *The Morality of Embryo Use.*

Facts

- Some ethicists believe that scientists should limit research to embryos resulting from spontaneous abortion (death of an embryo due to natural causes).

- According to a Gallup poll conducted shortly after Barack Obama lifted restrictions on ESC research in 2009, the majority of Americans feel that this research is morally permissible.

- Children born from unused IVF embryos that were given up for adoption have appeared before Congress to advocate for the rights of embryos.

- A number of religious groups, including the United Methodist Church and certain Jewish and Islamic groups, support ESC research if it has the potential to cure disease.

- The Roman Catholic Church, the Orthodox Church, and many conservative Protestant denominations believe an embryo has the status of a human being from the moment of conception and should therefore be protected.

Is Human Embryo Experimentation Necessary?

Many research scientists believe that human ESCs have the greatest potential to cure diseases because of their inherent ability to differentiate into almost any body tissue. However, few practical treatments have come from this research. US restrictions on funding for such research have also hampered progress. Indeed, the very lack of concrete treatments makes it even more difficult for scientists to obtain funding. Still, researchers are forging ahead in three key areas of investigation: research on human development, which in turn will foster knowledge about how diseases and disorders develop and progress; drug research and screening; and the development of novel treatments.

Toxicity Screening and New Drug Development

Though most people see the potential of stem cells in treating disease, many scientists are invested in this research because stem cells may aid in the testing procedures for drugs. Currently, new drugs must navigate lengthy trials, usually beginning with animal studies in which the drug under consideration must prove successful in order to move forward in the testing process. However, because significant differences are found in animal and human physiology, the drug must then be tested successfully on humans before the FDA will consider the drug effective and allow it to be manufactured and produced in the United States. Even with these safeguards, however, new drugs may still prove dangerous, and sometimes deadly. For example, Vioxx, a pain medication approved by the FDA in 1999 and thought to be free of dangerous side effects, was later found to cause heart damage. In fact, the drug was implicated in an estimated twenty-eight thousand heart attacks and sudden cardiac deaths before scientists determined that it caused serious heart risks.

These risks may be completely avoided with the use of ESCs instead of live subjects in the testing of drugs and chemicals. Scientists can grow pure samples of specific cell types in a petri dish, subject them to a variety of drugs and chemicals, and then measure the cell culture's response. With ESCs, scientists can quickly screen hundreds of thousands of chemical compounds to determine which are safe before they are used on human patients. In the case of Vioxx, for example, scientists would have been able to study cardiac cells in a petri dish and determine the relative safety of the drug far more easily than the current process allows. Doug Melton of the Harvard Stem Cell Institute states, "In the next decade, most advances will come from drugs that affect progression of disease. And we'll get there by using hES [human embryonic stem] cells as test beds for new therapeutics."[36]

Using an ESC's ability to take on the characteristics of any cell, scientists can cause an embryonic cell to differentiate into a diseased cell, such as a diseased liver or kidney cell, and then expose that cell to specific drug treatments. In this way researchers need not perform expensive animal or human test trials. Many researchers see this as one of the most exciting areas of stem cell research, predicting that the whole pharmaceutical process could be transformed from its current methods of using living organisms to a novel cellular approach in which no animal or human would ever again have to be exposed to the unknown risks of new drug trials. In congressional testimony

"In the next decade, most advances will come from drugs that affect progression of disease. And we'll get there by using hES [human embryonic stem] cells as test beds for new therapeutics."[36]

— Doug Melton, Harvard Stem Cell Institute researcher.

in 2010, Francis Collins, director of the NIH, described the process as a tool in fighting Lou Gehrig's disease (also known as amyotrophic lateral sclerosis, or ALS):

[Lou Gehrig's disease] is characterized by the progressive loss of motor neurons in the spinal cord which normally provide the connection between the brain and the muscles of the body. Now, ideally we would like to find a drug that stabilizes those human motor neurons against this kind of cell death, but how? Well, suppose you could test a library of hundreds of thousands of candidate drug compounds, knowing that somewhere in there, there might be one that would be valuable encouraging motor neurons to survive. . . . This is not a pipe dream. It is a reality. [A research laboratory] at Harvard is carrying out exactly this kind of experiment for ALS right now. The possibility that human embryonic stem cell research might one day enable us to identify a therapy for the disease that claimed the lives of so many . . . gives you some hope that this new application may provide answers that we desperately need.[37]

> "The possibility that human embryonic stem cell research might one day enable us to identify a therapy for the disease that claimed the lives of so many . . . gives you some hope that this new application may provide answers that we desperately need."[37]
>
> — Francis Collins, director of the NIH.

A Vehicle for Learning About Human Development

In addition to assisting in drug trials, stem cell research can also aid in the study of human development and, specifically, at what stages in development certain diseases and/or disorders develop. Traditionally, scientists study disease development in other organisms such as fruit flies, worms, or mice because such subjects have relatively short life spans when compared to humans, allowing their entire life cycle to be viewed quickly. However, translating information gathered from such organisms to humans requires further study and might not even be applicable to human patients. ESCs, however, are human cells, so results from tests on them are directly translatable to people. In addition, studying human ESCs offers a unique view of the earliest development of humans, giving insights

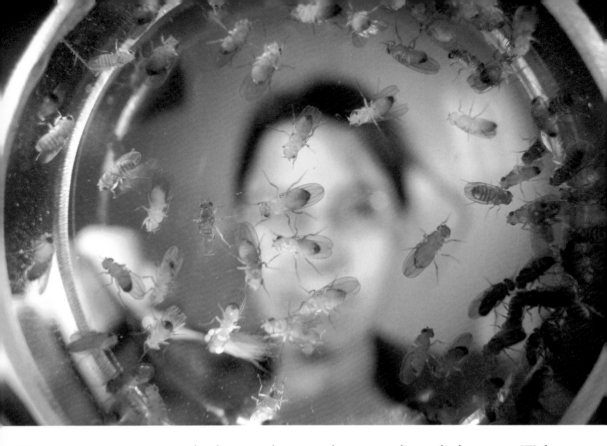

The relatively short life cycles of fruit flies (pictured) and other organisms make them good subjects for the study of how diseases develop even though the results are not always applicable to humans. Researchers say that similar studies with ESCs offer more relevant and potentially beneficial results.

into developmental activity that cannot be studied in utero. With stem cell research, scientists hope to understand how to prevent or treat medical problems in human reproduction, such as birth defects, miscarriages, and infertility. In short, ESCs can demonstrate how an undifferentiated group of cells turns into a highly complex human being—and what can go wrong along the way.

In his 2010 congressional testimony, Collins also spoke about the value of ESCs in helping scientists to understand the molecular pathways of disease:

For example, you might ask, what genes are expressed in human embryonic stem cells and how is that programming altered as these cells move down pathways to become blood cells, muscle cells, or brain cells, and how does that go awry in the presence of a disease mutation and cause an illness or a birth defect? One of the very best windows we have now into human development is through these human embryonic stem cells.[38]

Therefore, scientists can use these cells to study genetic conditions that involve chromosomal abnormalities, such as fragile X syndrome, a developmental disorder that affects mostly boys, and Rhett syndrome, a serious and debilitating brain disorder that affects primarily girls.

Human reproduction is not the only area in which stem cells can be used to discover the hidden beginnings of diseases and disorders. Researchers are using ESCs to grow vast quantities of heart tissues and other types of tissues to subject to various diseases. Such a large-scale study would be expensive, as well as difficult to test on a significant number of qualified patients. For this reason, the Coalition for the Advancement of Medical Research attests that

> hES cells are an unbeatable research tool to understand the body and what goes wrong in disease. Just like telescopes opened new vistas to distant galaxies, hES cells offer unprecedented access to the human body. Scientists are using hES cells to grow limitless quantities of various tissues, such as heart muscle cells. It will be a vast improvement over today's studies of the physiology of the human heart, which rely on limited biopsy samples from sick hearts.[39]

ESCs may also transform the way cancer is studied. Scientists can subject stem cells to various forms of cancer and learn more about how and why these diseases replicate in the body. Again, such research is possible without using a human subject.

Regenerative Medicine

As scientists continue to seek a clear understanding of the mechanisms of disease through research with stem cells, the end goal is to prevent, or at least slow the progression of, a variety of diseases and disorders. The most revolutionary proposals involve using stem cells in a process called cellular replacement therapy—essentially transplanting healthy cells derived from hES cells into patients to replace diseased or damage cells. The term *regenerative medicine* is used today to describe any treatment in which stem cells restore the function of damaged or diseased organs or tissues. To date, therapies using ESCs, while promising, are still in the very early

A Paralyzed Woman Speaks Out

Cody Unser, daughter of race car driver Al Unser Jr., was twelve years old when she developed a rare autoimmune disorder that damaged her spinal cord and left her paralyzed from the waist down. On September 16, 2010, she offered the following testimony before a Senate subcommittee hearing on the subject of stem cell research:

> Today I am a 23-year-old woman who has learned to adapt to life in a wheelchair and in a paralyzed body. . . . The first time hope actually meant something to me and became sort of my religion was when I saw what human embryonic stem cells can do. A year after I became paralyzed, my doctor and stem cell scientist, Doug Kerr, was at Johns Hopkins at the time, showed me a mouse that was once paralyzed and now can bear its weight and take steps. At that moment, I realized that this is science I couldn't ignore and it gave me a feeling of hope I wanted to fight for. Which brings me to another point. It's frustrating to hear critics of this research say this is a path we can't go down and adult stem cells hold just as much promise as embryonic stem cells do. Science is the pursuit of discovery and possibility. We should explore every opportunity and not count anything out because I can't wait. And I know millions of Americans now and in the future can't wait.

Cody Unser, "The Promise of Human Embryonic Stem Cells," US Senate Committee on Appropriations, Subcommittee on Labor, Health and Human Services, and Education, September 16, 2010. www.appropriations.senate.gov.

experimental stages and are not yet available to the public.

In fact, much of therapeutic stem cell research is still in its infancy, and researchers have a lot to learn before translating it into actual disease treatments. Years of intensive research will be needed to prove that ESCs can be effectively isolated and safely used. Cell development is very complex, and the growth of stem cell lines is difficult to control. For example, when cells are grown in a culture in the laboratory, they may lose some of the critical mechanisms that prohibit uncontrolled growth. This sometimes results in the growth of tumors, similar to the type of unrestricted growth seen in cancer cells. To use ESCs in human patients, scientists need to fully understand not just how to turn on cell reproduction but also how to turn it off. Furthermore, scientists must deal with a variety of risks, including a patient's immune response of rejecting ESCs grown in the laboratory. The latest research has revealed that just as in organ transplants, the recipient's immune system generates antibodies against foreign tissues or cells. Adult stem cells may prove more practical in such instances, as a patient's own cells can be harvested, cultivated, and reinjected. These cells are recognized by the body, and rejection is avoided.

Finally, scientists must develop a system of delivering the cells to the right part of the body and then devise ways to encourage those cells to integrate with other cells in the body. Commenting on this matter, the International Society for Stem Cell Research notes:

> One of the greatest barriers to the development of successful stem cell therapies is to get the cells to behave in the desired way. Also, once transplanted inside the body the cells need to integrate and function in concert with the body's other cells. For example, to treat many neurological conditions the cells we implant will need to grow into specific types of neurons, and to work they will also have to know which other neurons to make connections with and how to make these connections. We are still learning about how to direct stem cells to become the right cell type, to grow only as much as we need them to, and the best ways to transplant them. Discovering how to do all this will take time. *Be wary of claims that stem cells will somehow just know where to go and what to do to treat a specific condition.*[40]

Researchers may be able to make progress on this front soon. In 2010 the FDA approved the first human clinical trials using ESCs in the treatment of spinal cord injuries.

First Human Trials

Treating patients who have suffered paralysis from spinal cord injuries is one of the most exciting potential applications of ESCs. As previously noted, in October 2010 researchers from Geron Corporation in Menlo Park, California, administered ESCs to the first human patients. In this case researchers transplanted certain brain and spinal cord cells called oligodendrocytes that were derived from ESCs into individuals who had recently suffered spinal cord injury. Researchers hoped that the new cells would replicate within the body and restore some level of spinal cord function. As Geron's president, Thomas Okarma, said, "This marks the dawn of a new era in medical therapeutics. . . . This approach is one that reaches beyond pills and scalpels to achieve a new level of healing."[41] Before any definitive results could be gleaned, however, Geron announced that it was halting stem cell research to pursue cancer research, largely for financial reasons.

"One day, I looked down and I could see my watch. . . . I probably hadn't seen it in about a year and a half or two. And I could see. So that was exciting for me."[42]

— Sue Freeman, a patient in the first clinical trial using stem cells to treat macular degeneration.

Other studies using human subjects are under way, such as the work of the University of California and Advanced Cell Technology, the pair that is conducting two ongoing clinical trials that will assess the safety of using stem cell therapy to treat patients with macular degeneration. The disease attacks the center part of the retina, leaving people unable to see directly in front of them, though some peripheral vision remains. In this coordinated trial, researchers transplanted retinal cells developed from human ESCs into the eyes of two patients who suffer from different types of this progressive form of blindness. Preliminary reports released hint that the treatment is safe and effective, although it is far too early for any definitive conclusions to be drawn. However, after four months, the researchers found no signs of rejection, abnormal cell growth, or any other safety concerns.

Groundbreaking Results

Both patients in the University of California/Advanced Cell Technology trials experienced improvement in their vision—the first direct evidence that the transplantation of human ESCs into a human patient produced a marked, and verifiable, benefit. Before she had stem cells injected into her right eye to treat the macular degeneration that had left her legally blind, Sue Freeman, seventy-eight, could no longer recognize faces, read, cook, or go outside unassisted. Within six weeks of the procedure, she was performing such everyday tasks, which had been impossible for years. She said, "One day, I looked down and I could see my watch. . . . I probably hadn't seen it in about a year and a half or two. And I could see. So that was exciting for me. And I remember saying, 'Oh my goodness. I can see my watch. I can actually tell time.'"[42]

The second legally blind participant also showed improvement. A woman in her fifties, this patient remarked, "I sort of like woke up one morning and did realize that, 'Wow, you know, there is a difference between the two eyes now—they only worked on the left eye. . . . On the other side of the room I have some hand-carved furniture there. And I could actually see the detail on the carving, you know, on the other side of the room there, on things that I couldn't see from that distance before."[43]

While it is far too early to draw definitive conclusions, Steven D. Schwartz, a professor of ophthalmology at UCLA's Jules Stein Eye Institute and lead researcher of the trials, said, "I can't tell you how excited I am about this. . . . For these patients, the impact is enormous."[44] In a commentary that accompanied the report published in the British medical journal the *Lancet*, Anthony Atala of the Wake Forest Institute of the Wake Forest School of Medicine described the work as a turning point in ESC research. "The potential to use human embryonic derived cells with a therapeutic effect in patients is now finally realized,"[45] he said.

Other ESC research in progress focuses on diseases in animal models. Researchers hope to translate their results into human treatments while they work to overcome the obstacles that they face in controlling the growth and use of stem cells. Since animal

ESC research is less restricted than human ESC research, many more researchers have access to animal models and can conduct tests that might otherwise be prohibited.

Diabetes Research

One of the most promising pursuits in stem cell research focuses on diabetes, a leading cause of death in the United States. Diabetes is a disease that affects the body's ability to regulate sugar in the blood. Normally, when a person digests food, glucose (or sugar) enters the bloodstream. In response the pancreas releases the hor-

Alzheimer's Research Using Stem Cells

Alzheimer's disease is a progressive disease of the brain that causes the irreversible loss of brain neurons. Classic symptoms of Alzheimer's include loss of intellectual abilities, including memory and reasoning. It is incurable and eventually causes death. Research into this devastating disease poses unique challenges because Alzheimer's destroys many different types of cells in different regions of the brain. Many scientists believe that human ESCs, which could potentially develop into these different types of brain cells, are the perfect candidate for studying this complex disease.

In 2011 Northwestern Medicine researchers transformed an ESC into one of the neurons that dies in Alzheimer's disease and leads to memory loss. The ability to make these cells in the lab means that scientists can grow an almost unlimited supply for research into why this specific type of cell dies in Alzheimer's patients. Researchers can also quickly test tens of thousands of drugs to determine which ones could prevent these critical cells from dying. In this way scientists hope to one day stop the progression of the disease and to restore lost brain function.

mone insulin, which moves the glucose in the blood into the cells for energy. Type 1 diabetes develops when the body's immune system attacks these insulin-producing cells. Without enough insulin, the quantity of glucose in a person's blood can elevate to dangerous levels, wreaking havoc with a person's bodily functions, including circulation, heart function, and even the blood vessels in the eyes. Untreated, patients with diabetes may go blind, lose limbs to amputation due to poor blood circulation, or, most seriously, die from complications of the disease.

Patients with this disorder often must lose weight, restrict their diets, and take daily injections of insulin to regulate their blood-glucose levels. However, through stem cell research, scientists have demonstrated that certain types of pancreatic cells, called exocrine cells, can be reprogrammed to become beta cells, the type of cells that are destroyed in type 1 diabetes. Thus, scientists hope that stem cells might help create new insulin-producing cells, which would reduce the need for a diabetic's daily dose of insulin.

In a 2010 animal study, researchers at Stanford University cultured mouse ESCs that then developed into a tissue that produced insulin. When they grafted this special tissue into diabetic mice, the rodents produced enough insulin to sustain life. When researchers removed the tissue graft, the animals died from excess sugar in the blood. Robert Goldstein, chief scientific officer for the Juvenile Diabetes Research Foundation International, concluded, "The principle of being able to take embryonic stem cells and reverse diabetes is an extremely important observation."[46] Goldstein also commented, however, that it will be many years before this therapy can be used on humans.

> "The principle of being able to take embryonic stem cells and reverse diabetes is an extremely important observation."[46]
>
> — Robert Goldstein, chief scientific officer for the Juvenile Diabetes Research Foundation International.

Neurological Disorders

Researchers are also using stem cells to study neurological diseases such as Parkinson's disease, although it will also be years before stem cell therapies will be ready to treat human patients. Parkinson's is a progressive disorder that affects the brain and leads to uncontrolled tremors. As it progresses, Parkinson's also affects the brain, often leading to dementia similar to that seen in Alzheimer's disease. Parkinson's is caused by a disruption in the delivery system of the brain chemical dopamine; it is typically treated with drugs that activate dopamine receptors in the brain and control the symptoms in the initial stages of the disease. Investigators are looking at ways in which ESCs can be used to develop new neurons to produce dopamine in the body and alleviate symptoms. As James Thomson, who pioneered the development of the first human ESC lines in 1998, says, "I'd be very surprised if, during the course of my scientific career, the next 20 years, we don't have much better therapies for Parkinson's disease, based on the fact that we have these hESC-derived tissues in culture."[47]

Critics, however, have pointed out that despite such optimism, experiments have been problematic. In one experiment involving mice with Parkinson's, for example, 20 percent of the mice ended up with brain tumors after being treated with ESCs. Because of issues such as this, many opponents contend that human embry-

A patient who suffers from age-related macular degeneration is prepared for an antibody injection to treat vascular damage to the retina. Retinal cell transplants from embryonic stem cells might eventually replace this more traditional form of treatment.

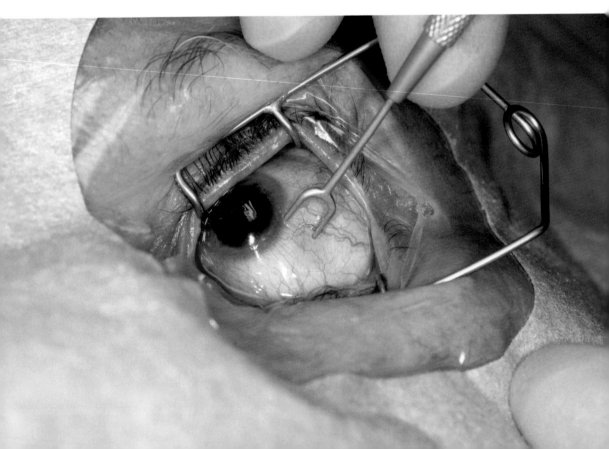

onic research requires so many years of additional research that the promise may never be fulfilled. British fertility expert Robert Winston remarks, "I am not entirely convinced that embryonic stem cells will, in my lifetime, and possibly anybody's lifetime for that matter, be holding quite the promise that we desperately hope they will."[48]

Another neurological disorder that scientists hope stem cells can help treat is Huntington's disease, which attacks the nervous system, causing loss of muscle coordination and cognitive ability and, eventually, death. The disease affects the levels of gamma-aminobutyric acid (GABA), a neurotransmitter that slows down the activity of nerve cells in the brain. When GABA neurons degrade, parts of the brain circuitry are disrupted, and patients lose muscle coordination and motor function. In a research study published in March 2012, neuroscientist Su-Chun Zhang and his colleagues at the University of Wisconsin discovered how to make GABA neurons from human ESCs, which they tested in a mouse model of Huntington's disease. To their astonishment, the cells integrated into the mouse brain, reestablished the broken neural circuits, and restored motor function. Researchers hope to one day use stem cell therapy to replace the damaged circuitry that causes diseases like Huntington's in humans; yet although the results are promising, much more research is needed before such therapies can be tested on patients.

"I am not entirely convinced that embryonic stem cells will, in my lifetime, and possibly anybody's lifetime for that matter, be holding quite the promise that we desperately hope they will."[48]

— British fertility expert Robert Winston.

A Vital Hope

Other disease research is even more preliminary. Stem cells could potentially repair damage in the brain and spinal cord through the regrowth of myelin, a fatty substance that encloses certain neurons and nerve fibers. Such regeneration could be used in patients suffering from brain injury as well. In all these and other areas of research, treatments are in their infant stages, and some are merely theoretical. To date, few concrete results have been produced, leading critics to argue that the therapeutic potential of stem cells has been greatly exaggerated.

For those suffering from debilitating illness, however, such research remains a vital hope. Patients argue that all research starts out as theoretical before it develops into real treatments. They hope for cures and worry that practical applications are not being hurried enough. Stem cell treatments might one day cure diseases, but until they proceed from theory to practice—if such applications are feasible at all—the promise remains just that.

Facts

- Before an ESC therapy can be used as treatment in the United States, the FDA requires at least two clinical trials to assess safety and effectiveness before considering approval of the technique.

- Researchers are using stem cells to create tests and potential treatments for developmental disorders such as autism.

- The seventh annual Wisconsin Stem Cell Symposium in 2012 brought together leaders in stem cell research to address a variety of brain and nervous system disorders.

- Researchers hope that ESCs may one day be used as a renewable source of healthy skin cells to treat burns and other medical problems that affect the skin.

- There is some evidence that ESCs can be programmed with the mutation that causes cystic fibrosis, a genetic disease that critically affects the lungs. This could enable scientists to study the progression of this serious disease.

What Are the Alternatives to Human Embryo Experimentation?

In the United States ESC research has been complicated by moral and ethical beliefs that prohibit its acceptance. In the face of such restrictions, scientists have been attempting to isolate and work with ASCs, which have many of the properties of ESCs but do not require the destruction of a human embryo. Because such research has been accepted on a broad scale, many scientists have made significant progress in some treatments.

Adult Stem Cells

Within days of fertilization, ESCs begin to differentiate into the many types of cells in the human body. As the embryo matures, a small number of undifferentiated cells remain in bone marrow, fat, skin, and other tissues. These cells, called adult stem cells, repair and maintain the tissue in which they are found. Scientists are learning to manipulate these cells to generate specific cell types that can be used to treat a variety of diseases and injuries.

Unlike ESCs, ASCs are capable of differentiating only into a small number of cells that develop into a specific organ or tissue. Most ASCs are multipotent cells because of their limited ability to differentiate; they often contrast with pluripotent ESCs that can differentiate into any cell type. Another limitation to ASCs is that they are extremely difficult to isolate, grow, and maintain in the laboratory. They will not reproduce indefinitely in culture, as do ESCs.

While these limitations render them unsuitable for certain types of research, the fact that culling ASCs does not result in the destruction of an embryo makes them a hugely attractive alternative to ESCs. Also, when the cells are derived from a person's own body, they do not generate an immune rejection. Today the mature stem cells culled from cartilage, blood, skin, and other tissues provide valuable insight into certain medical conditions and are used to treat a wide variety of diseases, including many cancers, cardiovascular disease, autoimmune disease, neural degenerative diseases, immunodeficiency disorders, and a variety of blood conditions.

Bone Marrow Transplants

Bone marrow transplantation is the most common example of a successful stem cell therapy using a patient's own stem cells. A bone marrow transplant uses blood stem cells that are present in bone marrow to treat a variety of diseases of the blood, including sickle-cell anemia and leukemia. These particular cells can be infused in the blood, and they will make their way to the bone marrow, where they replace the faulty cells. Doctors have been performing these procedures since 1956.

Advanced techniques for collecting these blood stem cells are currently in practice. Blood from an umbilical cord offers one of the richest sources of these particular cells. Cord cells can be extracted after the baby is born and stored in stem cell banks, which are similar to blood banks. If needed, these cells can be used later by the donor because they are a perfect genetic match. Other family members can receive treatment from these cells, too; although the more distant the relationship, the greater the likelihood the cells will be rejected. Even when they are not an exact genetic match, however, certain procedures will increase the chance that they will not be rejected.

A new program at the University of Virginia Health System has been collecting nonembryonic stem cells from donated umbilical cords and using the cells to treat leukemia, lymphoma,

The NIH Stance on Stem Cell Research

The current policy of the NIH is to pursue multiple lines of stem cell research. The organization contends that ASCs have potential weaknesses, such as DNA abnormalities, that may limit their usefulness, while human ESCs and induced pluripotent cells, which may have greater potential than ASCs, will require years of research before their full potential is unleashed. The NIH states:

> The development of stem cell lines that can produce many tissues of the human body is an important scientific breakthrough. This research has the potential to revolutionize the practice of medicine and improve the quality and length of life. Given the enormous promise of stem cell therapies for so many devastating diseases, NIH believes that it is important to simultaneously pursue all lines of research and search for the very best sources of these cells.

NIH Stem Cell Information, "Frequently Asked Questions," May 1, 2012. http://stemcells.nih.gov.

Hodgkin's disease, and other blood diseases. Doctors at the program performed two stem cell transplants on patients suffering from blood diseases in early 2012. The stem cells began producing new cells fourteen days after the transplant—twice as quickly as conventional bone marrow transplants. Although it is too early to know the results of such treatments, the initial findings are promising. The head of the program, stem cell expert Mary Laughlin, said an obstetrician told her, "Something thrown away in my OB [obstetrics] suite saves a life in your cancer suite."[49]

Cord blood has also shown promise in reducing the amount of insulin diabetes patients need to take. When a person has Type 1 diabetes, the body's own immune system attacks and destroys insulin-producing cells in the pancreas. In a small study performed at the University of Illinois–Chicago in January 2012, doctors attempted to reeducate diabetics' T cells, the white blood cells that help control the body's immune response, to reduce the system's attack on the pancreatic cells. Doctors separated a patient's own lymphocytes (immune cells that include T cells) and then cocultured them with stem cells from donor cord blood. The blood was circulated for two to three hours and then reinserted into the patient's own blood. Though the study was small (thirteen patients), all of the patients were able to reduce their insulin intake. Those with moderate diabetes were able to reduce their insulin intake by 38 percent, and those with severe diabetes were able to reduce their intake by 25 percent. Yong Zhao, who led the study, claims, "We also saw an improved autoimmune control in these patients. Stem Cell Educator therapy increased the percentage of regulatory T lymphocytes in the blood of people in the treatment group."[50]

Preventing Organ Transplant Rejection

This diabetic study produced some small success in suppressing the body's immune response. Doctors are experimenting with this same effect in hopes of reducing the body's rejection of organ transplants. Traditionally, patients undergoing a transplant must take immunosuppressive drugs to block the body's immune system from rejecting the new organ. These drugs are not without serious side effects, however, including reducing resistance to infections and the possibility of destroying the new organ. One study conducted by scientists from the Diabetes Research Institute at the Miller School of Medicine in the United States and a DRI Federation center at Xiamen University in China involved kidney transplant patients. In patients who had received kidney transplants to treat end-stage renal failure, stem cells were used along with traditional immunosuppressant drugs to see whether these individuals were better able to tolerate the new organs. After one year, patients who received the stem cells had a lower incidence of organ rejection, less risk from infection, and better overall kidney function. "This study represents a first, important step toward . . . strategies that will one day allow for transplantation without the need for life-long anti-rejection drugs,"[51] reports Camillo Ricordi, director of the University of Miami Diabetes Research Institute and Cell Transplant Center.

A similar study was conducted at the University of Louisville in Kentucky and the Northwestern Memorial Hospital in Chicago and involved eight kidney patients. Five of the eight patients were completely weaned off antirejection drugs within a year. One patient, forty-seven-year-old Lindsay Porter, claims, "I hear about

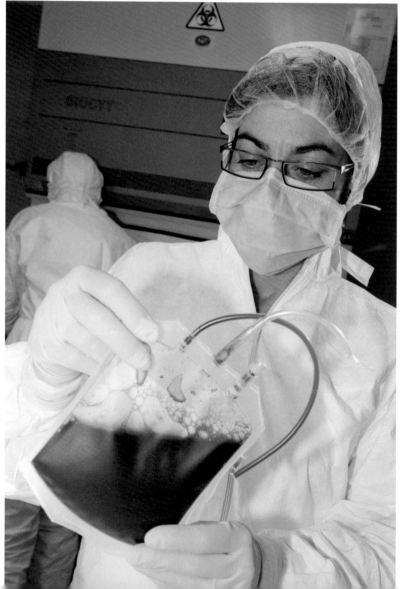

A laboratory technician manipulates a pouch filled with umbilical cord blood. Cord blood, a rich source of nonembryonic stem cells, offers promise for the treatment of leukemia, lymphoma, and other blood diseases.

the challenges recipients have to face with their medications and it is significant. . . . It's almost surreal when I think about it because I feel so healthy and normal."[52]

Jean Peduzzi-Nelson is a stem cell researcher—and an ardent supporter of ASC science—at Wayne State University in Michigan. At a 2010 hearing, Peduzzi-Nelson told members of Congress about patients who have benefited from ASC treatments, including a patient named Joe Davis Jr., who was born with severe sickle-cell anemia and treated with stem cells from his brother's umbilical cord blood. Peduzzi-Nelson stated:

> Sickle cell anemia is a blood disease that affects 1/500 African Americans. The doctors thought that Joe might not live to see his teens. When Joe was 2 years old in 2002, he received a transplant of stem cells from his younger brother's umbilical cord. Joe no longer has sickle cell anemia. So, where are we now? About 72,000 people in the US have sickle cell anemia that causes pain, chronic tiredness from anemia and severe infections, usually beginning when they are babies. . . . It would be great if we could have everyone with sickle cell anemia treated.[53]

As proof of the efficacy of ASCs, Peduzzi-Nelson cites a number of published studies that back up her position, such as a 2009 study in the *New England Journal of Medicine*, in which ten adults with sickle-cell anemia were treated with ASCs from a sibling. Out of these ten patients, nine no longer had symptoms of the disease at the conclusion of the study.

Birth Defects and Heart Disease

ASCs are being used in trials to treat other health issues, such as birth defects. Angela Irizarry, for example, is a young child who was born with hypoplastic left heart syndrome, which affects three thousand newborns every year in the United States. Children born with the condition have just one pumping chamber in their heart instead of two, which deprives the body of sufficient oxygen. Without surgery, 70 percent of affected children die from the disease before their first birthday. Traditional treatment for the disease involves implanting a synthetic blood vessel to reroute blood directly to the lungs, allowing the heart's existing pumping chamber to pump blood just to the body. The procedure works but is often prone to clotting and infection. As a child with this condition grows, he or she needs additional surgery to take on the increasing demands of a growing body. In the first stem cell therapy for the disorder, doctors implanted in Angela's chest a temporary, bioabsorbable tube that contained stem cells harvested from Angela's bone marrow. The tube has since dissolved and has left a conduit in its place that functions like a blood vessel. Pediatric surgeon Christopher Breuer, who led the procedure, says, "We're making a blood vessel where there wasn't one. . . . We're inducing regeneration."[54] The results in Angela were marked; for the first time in her life, she had the energy level of a normal child her age. As her father says, "It's a huge difference. . . . It's like going from a four-cylinder to an eight-cylinder car in one operation."[55]

"It's not hype, it is really hope. . . . I think that stem cells will likely become a routine part of the treatment of cardiovascular disease in the next few years."[56]

— Roberto Bolli, chief cardiologist at the University of Louisville.

Other cardiac specialists are developing their own treatments using ASCs. Roberto Bolli, chief cardiologist at the University of Louisville, has used ASCs in treating patients who have experienced heart failure. He believes such treatment has tremendous potential. "It's not hype, it is really hope," he says. "I think that stem cells will likely become a routine part of the treatment of cardiovascular disease in the next few years."[56]

Breakthroughs Continue

The involvement of stem cells in generating new tissue is part of much new research both in the United States and internationally. In Germany, for example, a cancer victim whose jaw had been removed grew new bone tissue after having his own stem cells, taken from his bone marrow, transplanted.

One of the difficult obstacles in stem cell regeneration therapy has been to get stem cells to migrate to specific targets in the body and start regenerating where they are needed. Researchers at the University of California–Davis Health System have made a breakthrough in this area by injecting a molecule into the bloodstream that tells the body's stem cells to travel to the surface of bones to start regenerating bone formation and strength. The study was performed on mice with osteoporosis (a bone disease that increases the risk of fractures) whose bodies began to regenerate the damaged bone. Scientists hope to use the molecule in a human trial soon. Wei Yao, who headed the study, claims, "Finding a molecule that attaches to stem cells and guides them to the targets we need is a real breakthrough."[57] While the breakthrough has the potential to help the 4 million Americans, mostly women, who have osteoporosis, similar technology could induce stem cells to migrate to other parts of the body where they are needed to regenerate specific areas.

The use of ASCs to treat patients with spinal cord injury is another promising area of research. At the 2010 congressional hearing, Peduzzi-Nelson related the story of a patient named Silvio, who was treated by a group of Portuguese doctors led by Carlos Lima:

> Silvio had a [Grade A] spinal cord injury at the base of his neck. . . . Grade A is considered the worst, which indicates a "complete" spinal cord injury where no motor or sensory function is preserved in the sacral segments S4-S5. Silvio was left with no movement of his legs and minimal movement of his fingers. At 2 years after injury, he received his own adult stem cells and partial scar removal after intensive rehab failed to lead to an improvement.

> Today he can maintain standing position and wave without help. With a walker and short braces, he can walk over 30 feet without anyone helping him. He can now move his fingers, which he could not do before.[58]

Many believe that these exciting treatments mean that ESCs may never have to be used. Doctor Mary L. Davenport argues that "scientists know that claims of imminent cures of disease using embryonic stem cells are junk science, whereas progress in adult stem cell research has been nothing short of spectacular."[59] Some

"Finding a molecule that attaches to stem cells and guides them to the targets we need is a real breakthrough."[57]

— Wei Yao, researcher at the University of California–Davis Health System.

insiders caution, though, that even treatments using a patient's own stem cells are not necessarily safe. The International Society for Stem Cell Research reports:

> While your own cells are less likely to be rejected by your immune system, this does not necessarily mean the cells are safe to use as a therapeutic treatment. The methods used to isolate, modify, grow or transplant the cells may alter the cells, could cause infection or introduce other unknown risks. Transplanting cells into a different part of the body than they originated from may have unforeseen risk, complications or unpredictable outcomes.[60]

Proponents of ESCs are also quick to point out that only ESCs can become any type of human cell and therefore carry the greatest potential to treat a wide spectrum of diseases and disorders. The National Cancer Institute notes that "embryonic stem cells hold far more potential than adult cells" when it comes to research, because embryonic cells "can change into more tissue types and replicate indefinitely, two properties not generally shown with adult cells."[61]

The debate over ESCs versus ASCs, however, may be overshadowed by even newer and more experimental research that involves creating customized stem cells to treat disease.

"While your own cells are less likely to be rejected by your immune system, this does not necessarily mean the cells are safe to use as a therapeutic treatment."[60]

— International Society for Stem Cell Research.

Induced Pluripotent Stem Cells

Induced pluripotent stem cells (iPSCs) are another type of stem cells. These are non-pluripotent cells that were genetically manipulated to become pluripotent and therefore give rise to all cell types in the human body. These cells were first produced in 2007 when researchers inserted genetic instructions into skin cells, thereby reprogramming them to an unspecialized state similar to that of ESCs. In addition to being able to form all cell types in the human body and divide indefinitely, these cells represent a major breakthrough in the development of treatments for a variety of conditions because they are derived from the patient and therefore overcome the problems of immune rejection.

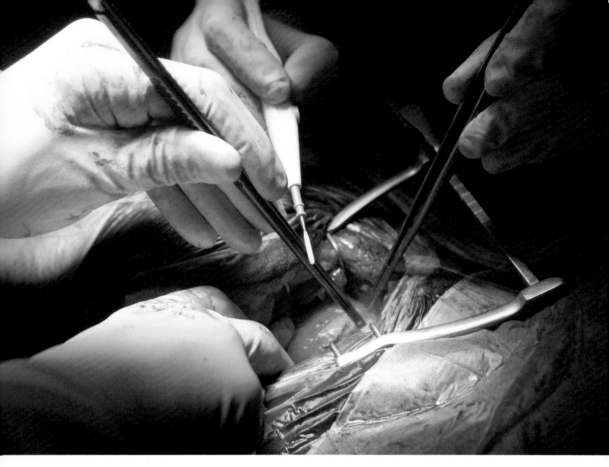

Surgeons perform a kidney transplant. New research suggests that adult stem cells might help reduce the incidence of organ rejection and infection in kidney transplant patients.

Another major attribute of iPSCs is that they are created from adult cells, so no major ethical concerns are associated with their use. Many people think that funds currently being used to research ESCs should be diverted instead to these less controversial and, to some, more promising sources of stem cells.

According to the International Society for Stem Cell Research, a major advantage of these cells is that "they can be grown and expanded indefinitely in the laboratory. Therefore, in contrast to adult stem cells, cell number will be less of a limiting factor. Another advantage is that given their very broad potential, several cell types that are present in an organ might be generated. Sophisticated tissue engineering approaches are therefore being developed to reconstruct organs in the lab."[62] The hope for these cells is to differentiate them in a dish into different tissues, such as nerve cells for a patient with Parkinson's, and then study them to devise a custom treatment for the patient. But this is still years away.

First, scientists would have to take such cells and cure the genetic defects within them before hoping to reinject them into a patient as a treatment.

iPSCs were used to cure mice with sickle-cell anemia in a study in 2007. Scientists removed some skin cells from the mice, and then turned those cells into iPSCs. Scientists then snipped out the DNA pieces that cause sickle-cell anemia and filled those gaps of DNA with bits of DNA bearing the proper code. Finally, scientists took those cells and mutated them to mature into bone marrow cells. When the mice were reinjected with the corrected bone marrow cells, their blood cells began producing new cells free of the sickle cells. George Q. Daley, a stem cell researcher at Children's Hospital Boston, says, "I think it is a really exciting proof-of-principle that clinical applications of iPS cells are technically feasible."[63]

According to the Coalition for the Advancement of Medical Research, iPSCs may also be used

> to personalize cancer therapies. Before a cancer patient takes a chemotherapy regimen that is extremely toxic, doctors could take a skin cell from the patient, and through the iPS process, create liver cells and heart cells. The chemotherapy could be tested first on those patients' "own" cells. A new drug regimen would only be given to the patient after it is clear that the drugs will kill the cancer, not the patient.[64]

Research with iPSCs is still preliminary, however, and many fundamental questions about iPSC safety and utility remain unanswered. For example, while iPSCs and ESCs share many characteristics, researchers note that there are subtle but important differences between the two. Furthermore, scientists must insert up to four genes into mature cells such as skin cells to render them pluripotent, and the consequences of this genetic manipulation are not fully understood. Researchers continue to manipulate these cells with different combinations of genes and different methods of inserting them as they ascertain how and if these procedures alter the cell in unintended ways. One of the most pressing problems, for example, is that iPSCs have formed tumors when transplanted into mice. As scientists work out these and other safety

Stem Cell Tourism

Because a number of ASC treatments are now being used to treat patients, many people advocate global regulations not only for research, but also for stem cell treatment. Today many patients travel abroad for novel stem cell therapies that are not available in the United States. Many experts warn against this so-called stem cell tourism, claiming that patients need to be cautious about the claims made by unscrupulous doctors hoping to profit from patients desperate to find cures. As New York State Stem Cell Science explains:

> While many clinics advertise stem cell cures for many different diseases, clinical trials on the use of stem cells are very limited. Most of the success stories reported in the news and on the internet are anecdotal accounts. The reports on the success of such treatments cannot replace large-scale, rigorously controlled clinical trials to prove both the safety and efficacy of treatments. Additionally, the people running such clinics and profiting from them are the same people declaring them to be safe and successful, presenting potential conflicts of interest.

New York State Stem Cell Science, "Stem Cell Science Frequently Asked Questions," 2012. http:// stemcell.ny.gov.

concerns, many believe that such work cannot and should not replace research into ESCs. ESC research remains crucial to research pertaining to all types of stem cells. According to the Coalition for the Advancement of Medical Research:

> Access to hES cells is crucial to continued progress. These pluripotent cells that can self-renew are an unmatched

research tool for understanding the body and what goes wrong in disease. Researchers refer to them as "the gold standard" because these are the cells with the greatest potential for making any cell type in the body. Study of these cells has led to the development of other potential sources of self-renewing cells, such as the reprogramming of adult skin cells to make induced pluripotent stem (iPS) cells. The ability to make iPS cells demonstrates the power of hES cell research to transform science and create new medical opportunities.[65]

Most researchers argue that the study of any one of these cells—embryonic stem cells, adult stem cells, and induced pluripotent stem cells—is still too new to decide that one can completely replace the other. Much of the research remains theoretical.

Therapeutic Cloning

Another alternative to traditional ESCs are stem cells created through somatic cell nuclear transfer (SCNT). In this procedure a somatic cell—any cell from the human body aside from the sperm or egg—is transferred into a human egg from which the nucleus—containing the cell's DNA—has been removed. The egg is manipulated to develop as though it had been fertilized with sperm. It is able to keep dividing until it is a blastocyst with about 150 cells. ESCs can be culled from this blastocyst. A major benefit of SCNT is that the stem cells derived from this technique are genetically identical to the patient that donated the body cell. They can also produce all cell types and are relatively easy to grow and maintain in the laboratory.

This technique is called therapeutic cloning because, although these types of cells have no practical application to date, they could one day be used in therapy. Researchers have used nuclear transfer techniques in a number of animals. In 2007 researchers at the Oregon National Primate Research Center established the first successful stem cell line after nuclear transfer in a primate, fostering enthusiasm that this technique could be feasible with humans. In 2011 scientists at the New York Stem Cell Foundation Laboratory used cloning technology to add the nuclei of adult skin cells from patients with type 1 diabetes to an unfertilized adult human egg cell to create a developing embryo—and ESCs. Although the embryos were not true clones because scientists left some of the egg's DNA intact, it brings science one step closer to successful therapeutic cloning.

In addition to technical hurdles, therapeutic cloning presents many of the same ethical concerns as ESC research because an embryo is destroyed when the stem cells are extracted. Many scientists counter that since the human blastocysts are created asexually, they would have little if any potential to be born alive (for the same reasons scientists have so many problems cloning animals). Because they cannot become human beings, they should not present the same ethical concerns as other embryos. Many critics take no comfort in this type of logic, however, arguing that creating human life in a test tube for the express purpose of using it in a scientific experiment is horrendously wrong. And, because the technique is basically the same technique used in reproductive cloning, scientists could one day clone live human beings. This slippery slope to creating life in a test tube is unacceptable to many people.

The technique also requires the donation of large numbers of human eggs. SCNT is so difficult—the egg with the somatic material is extremely unstable—that many attempts are required to produce even one viable egg. Some estimate that several hundred human eggs would be needed to cull enough stem cells for a single therapeutic application. How scientists would obtain these eggs, and the sheer number that would be destroyed in the process, bothers many ethicists.

In light of these issues, iPSCs seem a far less complicated ethical choice, since they provide an unlimited supply of undifferentiated cells without any ethical concerns. The International Society for Stem Cell Research sums up some of the most prominent issues concerning the use of iPSCs:

Why use these? First, these cells could provide a powerful new tool for studying the basis of human disease and for

"[Induced pluripotent stem cells] could provide a powerful new tool for studying the basis of human disease and for discovering new drugs."[66]

— International Society for Stem Cell Research.

discovering new drugs. Second, the resulting embryonic stem cells could be developed into mature cell types. After transplantation into the original donor, these would be recognized as "self," thereby avoiding the problems of rejection and immunosuppression that occur with transplants from unrelated donors. It is possible however that the recent development of iPS cells will supersede the use of somatic nuclear transfer as it is technically easier and does not require the use of eggs, avoiding issues with human egg procurement.[66]

Currently, investigation into all cell types continues as scientists try to achieve new treatments while adhering to the ethical construct around the legislation regarding ESCs. As new technologies for treating complex diseases make progress, however, patient lobbies will also weigh in on the discussion.

Facts

- In 2011 scientists at Stanford University demonstrated that iPSCs could be manipulated to carry a genetic mutation that causes the connective-tissue disease Marfan syndrome; this enables scientists to study the inherited disorder.

- As reported in the *Journal of Cranio-Maxillofacial Surgery* in 2004, ASCs helped repair skull damage in a seven-year-old girl.

- Victims of Iraqi mustard gas attacks who were left blind regained their eyesight following ASC transplants.

- Since 2007, veterinarians at Vet-Stem in San Diego, California, have treated over seven thousand arthritic horses and dogs with fat-derived stem cells.

- In a study at the Washington Center for Pain Management, ASCs derived from bone marrow will be injected into subjects with chronic back pain to ascertain whether this procedure may offer an alternative to back surgery.

- A 2012 study at the Georgia Health Sciences University will assess whether the transfusion of ASCs after a stroke will improve the chances that patients will recover.

How Should Human Embryo Experimentation Be Funded?

Human embryo experimentation has been subject to intense scrutiny and regulated by strict rules that govern its use. As more is known about its possibilities to treat disease and to reveal more information about human health and development, the ways it should be funded and regulated continue to cause heated debate.

Federal Funding

Supporters argue that restrictions on human embryo experimentation should be eased. They insist the federal government should fund embryo research that can lead to treatments that will save lives. When George W. Bush signed an executive mandate in 2001 that restricted federal funding to research on ESC lines already in existence and excluded research that destroys embryos, many felt he dealt a crippling blow to research. It was not until 2009 that the Bush-era stem cell policies were overturned when Barack Obama signed Executive Order 13505: Removing Barriers to Responsible Scientific Research Involving Human Stem Cells, which states that the government may support and conduct responsible and worthy human ESC research.

Obama's change in policy—his order permits funding of research on new cell lines created after 2001 and on cell lines created from embryos left over from reproductive procedures—opened a

Stem Cell Guidelines

In general, institutions that receive funding for stem cell research must adhere to the guidelines of the funding agency. Guidelines have been developed by the NIH, the National Academies, and the International Society for Stem Cell Research. In April 2005, for example, the National Academies released its Guidelines for Human Embryonic Stem Cell Research, which requires ethical review of the research by an Embryonic Stem Cell Research Oversight committee that includes not only scientists and doctors but also ethicists and community members. The guidelines were amended in 2010 to reflect Barack Obama's 2009 policy changes that permit research with human embryos. The amended guidelines exhort scientific investigators and their institutions to

> bear the ultimate responsibility for ensuring that they conduct themselves in accordance with professional standards and with integrity. In particular, people whose research involves hES cells should work closely with oversight bodies, demonstrate respect for the autonomy and privacy of those who donate gametes [sperm or eggs], morulae [embryos at an early stage of development], blastocysts, or somatic cells and be sensitive to public concerns about research that involves human embryos.

National Academies, *Final Report of the National Academies' Human Embryonic Stem Cell Research Advisory Committee and 2010 Amendments to the National Academies' Guidelines for Human Embryonic Stem Cell Research.* Washington, DC: National Academies Press, 2010. p. 23.

floodgate of new research. Many in the scientific community considered this a critical step in finding cutting-edge cures that could save the lives of millions of people suffering from heart disease, cancer, and other debilitating conditions.

Advocates believe that one of the reasons Obama's policies will have such a huge impact is that, as of 2012, 136 human ESC lines are eligible for federal money. In contrast, the Bush administration had authorized 60 existing ESC lines for research. However, only about 22 of these were useful to researchers because many of the cell lines lacked genetic diversity, had chromosomal abnormalities, or presented other problems. In short, cells from these preexisting lines did not represent the full range of human genetic diversity. Yet what many see as a reasonable compromise, others see as an attack on human life and want legislation that repeals Obama's order.

Indeed, religious figures and other opponents who believe that the government should not fund research that is morally questionable have sharply criticized Obama for lifting constraints on embryonic research. The moral issue has generated contentious political debate at a national level. Many liberal politicians favor funding, but the issue remains divisive among conservatives. Former first lady Nancy Reagan, who watched her husband, former Republican president Ronald Reagan, succumb to Alzheimer's disease, has become a vocal proponent of using federal funds for stem cell research. She says:

> I'm very grateful that President Obama has lifted the restrictions on federal funding for embryonic stem cell research. These new rules will now make it possible for scientists to move forward. I urge researchers to make use of the opportunities that are available to them and to do all they can to fulfill the promise that stem cell research offers.
>
> Countless people, suffering from many different diseases, stand to benefit from the answers stem cell research can provide. We owe it to ourselves and to our children to do everything in our power to find cures for these diseases—and soon. As I've said before, time is short, and life is precious.[67]

Yet another viewpoint from the Republican Party is voiced by John Boehner, Speaker of the House of Representatives, who criticized Obama's decision to use federal funds for ESC research. Boehner attests:

> I fully support stem cell research, but I draw the line at taxpayer-funded research that requires the destruction of human embryos, and millions of Americans feel similarly. As we move forward, I am hopeful that the President will re-evaluate this and other controversial decisions that put government at odds with the sanctity of human life. Non-embryonic stem cell research is not only showing great promise in the laboratory, but its applications are already being used to treat scores of diseases and medical conditions. Indeed, science and respect for human life can coexist. Politicians in Washington would be well-served to recognize this fact before they ask taxpayers to subsidize the destruction of innocent human life simply to advance a particular agenda.[68]

"I fully support stem cell research, but I draw the line at taxpayer-funded research that requires the destruction of human embryos, and millions of Americans feel similarly."[68]

— Speaker of the US House of Representatives John Boehner.

Like Boehner, Virginia representative Randy Forbes also contends that government funding should support research that will further the science of nonembryonic stem cells. Speaking out against the inauguration of Executive Order 13505, Forbes proclaimed, "The President's action today ignores the incredible advances we have seen in adult stem cell treatments, including the multitude of studies documenting patients who have been treated for Parkinson's disease, type 1 diabetes, Alzheimer's disease, cancer and other diseases through adult stem cells."[69]

Interestingly, Senator Orrin Hatch of Utah, who is a vocal abortion opponent, Mormon, and conservative Republican, lobbied for legislation to support ESC research. Hatch says, "Abortion destroys life; this is about saving lives." He also opined that "the most pro-life position would be to help people who suffer from these maladies."[70]

In this political climate Obama's order will likely continue to be challenged in the US court system. For example, in 2010 a judge temporarily blocked the use of federal funds for ESC research. The judge ruled in a pending lawsuit brought by a group of scientists who claimed that funding ESC research would compete with funding of ASC research and violate the Dickey-Wicker Amendment. Although a federal judge dismissed the case and ruled in the government's favor, the case foreshadows the legal challenges ahead.

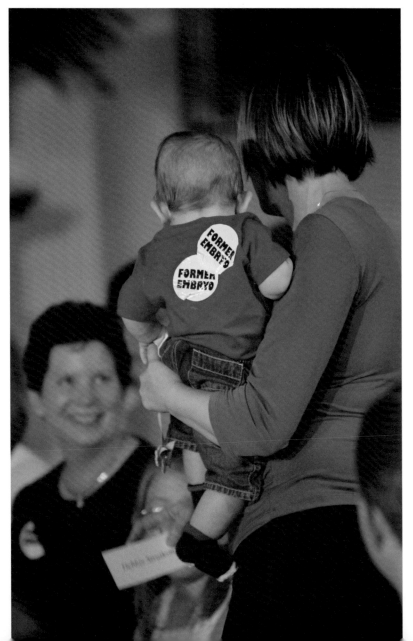

Families who oppose federal funding for any research that results in the destruction of human embryos meet with President George W. Bush in 2005. One woman carries a baby whose shirt reads, "Former Embryo."

State Funding

Traditionally, the federal government has been a major source of funding for biomedical research through grants from the NIH. But Bush's decision in 2001 to limit federal funding to ESC lines already in existence paved the way for state governments to establish and fund stem cell research programs. In 2004 New Jersey became the first state to commit state money—$9.5 million—to ESC research. Later the same year California voters approved Proposition 71, which allocated $3 billion to fund adult and ESC research over the subsequent ten years. Since then many states have struggled over whether to follow suit. Leon Rosenberg, a professor of molecular biology and public affairs at Princeton University, said of this unusual action: "It is an unprecedented foray by states into the federal terrain. Never before have the states stepped in to fund life sciences."[71] Like New Jersey and California, a number of other states have decided that this is a science worth pursuing. States attempting to encourage such research through funding programs include Connecticut, Illinois, Maryland, New York, and Wisconsin, although the specific policies vary from state to state. In California, for example, Proposition 71 led to the establishment of the California Institute for Regenerative Medicine, a state research institute that oversees funding of ESC research. The institute claims it funds "all phases of research from basic science that produces the breakthrough ideas all the way through filing paperwork to begin clinical trials."[72] The institute is currently funding research to develop therapies for blood diseases such as sickle-cell anemia, certain cancers, eye diseases, and a broad range of neurological disorders and other ailments. Similarly, the state of New York created a publicly funded program, New York State Stem Cell Science, which supports research related to stem cells at academic institutions, research institutions, and medical centers located in New York State.

Many think that such state funding means that cutting-edge and potentially lifesaving research will not be limited by political whims. Former New Jersey governor Richard Cody argues that his state and others are simply trying to help people through promising research. He explains:

A lot of people have been asking . . . "Why should the state support stem cell research?" It is full of hope, but it is controversial, and there are no guarantees. I believe that as a society and a government, we have an obligation to help those among us who are suffering. If we have an opportunity to save lives we must pursue it. And stem cell research is that opportunity. It is our best hope for the grandmother who is slowly slipping away to Alzheimer's or the retiree whose golden years are tortured by Parkinson's or the high school athlete who is paralyzed by a spinal cord injury.[73]

Despite such claims, some people question whether states should be filling a role traditionally assumed by the federal government. Critics argue that states cannot provide the same regulatory oversight, for example, that the federal government provides. Some researchers fear that states may not have the experience to fund the most worthy research projects or the finances and political stamina to fund research over decades of experimentation.

In addition, some politically conservative states have used the issue of human embryo research to legislate their own bans. Louisiana and South Dakota have passed laws, for example, making it illegal to perform research that results in the destruction of human embryos. Still other states, such as Missouri and Iowa, have declared that ESC research is legal, yet offer no funding.

Some states with restrictive laws or bans on this type of research are being persuaded to soften their moral stance. These state governments are finding that voters commonly support research that benefits humanity or at least holds the potential to do so. In November 2008 Michigan voters approved a ballot proposal that created a constitutional amendment to ease the strict prohibitions in the state, electing to allow scientific institutions to use embryos donated by couples undergoing fertility treatments to derive new stem cell lines. The changes to Michigan law have enabled researchers to apply for state government funding as they search

"[ESC research] is our best hope for the grandmother who is slowly slipping away to Alzheimer's or the retiree whose golden years are tortured by Parkinson's or the high school athlete who is paralyzed by a spinal cord injury."[73]

— Richard Cody, former governor of New Jersey.

for new cures. Since then the University of Michigan has emerged as a leader in ESC research. Scientists there have created several new stem cell lines that uniquely carry genetic defects. Using these lines, the scientists hope to uncover what goes wrong in these cells and to ascertain what drugs can treat these diseased or defective cells. This position of leadership could not have been achieved without the will of the people to overturn established policies.

Private Organizations

Because the federal government permits research even if it does not fund it, universities, biotech companies, and other private organizations are free to pursue ESC programs, often with their own resources. Unless a specific state law prohibits it, many private companies are forging ahead, sometimes without government funding or with a combination of government and private funding. For example, much of the research leading to the first clinical trial using human ESCs at Geron Corporation was funded not by the federal government but by the biotech company itself. The

A researcher who is affiliated with the California Institute for Regenerative Medicine works with stem cells in her lab. Several states have created programs to encourage continued work in cutting-edge stem cell technologies.

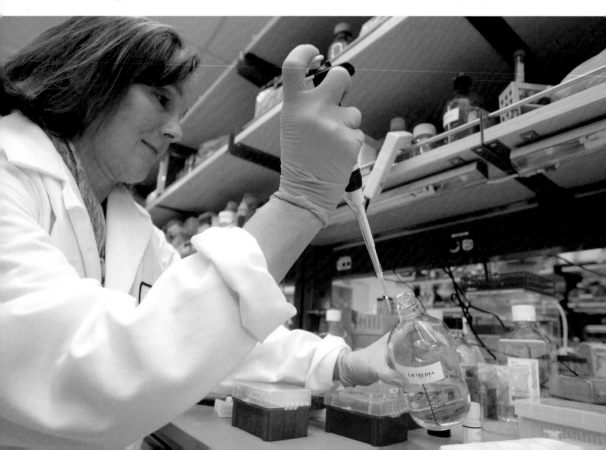

company also received a large grant from the California Institute for Regenerative Medicine. When the research was cut short, Geron cited financial difficulties. Many proponents believe this illustrates the many hazards to private funding that scientists do not experience when federal funds support a research goal.

Even with such drawbacks, many scientists prefer private funding. As Sigrid Fry-Revere, president of the Center for Ethical Solutions, writes:

> The great advantage of private funding is that it allows research to proceed even—especially—when it is politically touchy. When the federal government refused to fund in-vitro fertilization research in the mid-1970s, critics cried that the U.S. would fall behind, that there would be a brain drain, and that infertile couples would suffer. None of these dire predictions came true. Instead, the research proceeded privately and today reproductive technologies—IVF and related technologies for humans and animals—represent a $16 billion a year industry in the U.S. alone.[74]

Whereas scientists who wish to conduct stem cell research might find it difficult to compete for scarce government funds, many are successful in soliciting private donations. For example, the Harvard Stem Cell Institute, which conducts research into stem cell therapies for diabetes, cancer, cardiovascular disease, and other conditions, is supported almost entirely by private philanthropic donations, as are many other research institutes affiliated with universities.

Today many organizations continue to receive both private and government donations, but because restrictions remain on what research is eligible for federal funding—only discarded embryos from reproductive clinics that have the donor's consent qualify for funding—this can present challenges. For example, many research organizations conduct different types of research concurrently—some that is eligible for federal or state funding and some that is not. In this scenario, equipment and facilities must sometimes be

"The great advantage of private funding is that it allows research to proceed even—especially—when it is politically touchy."[74]

— Sigrid Fry-Revere, founder and president of the Center for Ethical Solutions.

Obama Defends His Stance

When Barack Obama signed the executive order to lift the ban on federal funding for stem cell research, he stated:

> The full promise of stem cell research remains unknown, and it should not be overstated. But scientists believe these tiny cells may have the potential to help us understand, and possibly cure, some of our most devastating diseases and conditions. To regenerate a severed spinal cord and lift someone from a wheelchair. To spur insulin production and spare a child from a lifetime of needles. To treat Parkinson's, cancer, heart disease and others that affect millions of Americans and the people who love them.
>
> But that potential would not reveal itself on its own. Medical miracles do not happen simply by accident. They result from painstaking and costly research—from years of lonely trial and error, much of which never bears fruit—and from a government willing to support that work. From life-saving vaccines, to pioneering cancer treatments, to the sequencing of the human genome—that is the story of scientific progress in America. When government fails to make these investments, opportunities are missed. Promising avenues go unexplored. Some of our best scientists leave for other countries that will sponsor their work. And those countries may surge ahead of ours in the advances that transform our lives.

Barack Obama, "Remarks of President Barack Obama—as Prepared for Delivery: Signing of Stem Cell Executive Order and Scientific Integrity Presidential Memorandum," White House, March 9, 2009. www.whitehouse.gov.

duplicated so that federal funds do not apply to research not allowed under Obama's order.

In addition, while the Harvard Stem Cell Institute and other well-established entities are able to garner generous charitable donations, others have problems soliciting adequate funding. For these and other reasons, many wish that organizations that have a vested interest in eradicating and treating a variety of diseases—such as the American Cancer Society, the American Heart Association, or Susan G. Komen for the Cure, which funds breast cancer research—should step forward and fund stem cell research. Says George Q. Daley, a stem cell researcher at Harvard University, "Funding science is supposed to be based on merit. . . . Scientific funding should support the best ideas. And if someone has a brilliant idea relevant to breast cancer research or heart disease that uses human embryonic stem cells, it'd be a huge lost opportunity to have one of these foundations refuse to fund it."[75]

Rose Marie Robertson, chief science officer at the American Heart Association, acknowledges that ESC research could lead to revolutionary treatments for heart disease. At the same time, she explains that the subject is so politically charged that the organization, which itself relies on charitable donations, would not supply funds. "There are people who have varying views in terms of whether they find this personally or ethically, or from a religious perspective, something that is reasonable," she claims. "If, in fact, donors chose not to support the heart association because of a particular view in terms of human-embryonic-stem-cell research that would be really harmful."[76]

Clearly, funding for human ESC research is complicated by the fact that many find the destruction of a human embryo unacceptable and do not want the federal government to use taxpayer money to pursue it. As it stands, the federal government helps fund many important research projects each year, and scientists must be creative when they need to find other means of funding. Yet in some states, voters are showing their support for such research and supplanting federal restrictions by voting to release state monies for funding. It appears that, like many avenues of scientific inquiry, the federal government cannot prevent scientists from pursuing their goals.

Facts

- So that research is not duplicated across states, the Interstate Alliance on Stem Cell Research works to foster interstate collaboration on all forms of stem cell research and promote the efficient use of public funds.

- Since 2005 the Starr Foundation, one of the largest private foundations supporting education and medicine, has awarded over $50 million for human ESC research at medical institutions in New York City.

- In 2001 the Johns Hopkins University in Maryland launched its Institute for Cell Engineering, which conducts ESC research, after an anonymous donor gave the university $58.5 million.

- In 2011 the California Institute for Regenerative Medicine lent $25 million to Geron Corporation to support the nation's first clinical trial involving ESCs.

- Many countries, including Australia, Brazil, Canada, France, and Spain, allow ESC research, some of which is funded by the European Union.

Source Notes

Introduction: A Cautionary Tale

1. Kazuo Ishiguro, *Never Let Me Go*. New York: Vintage, 2005, p. 286.
2. Kristen K. Intemann and Inmaculada de Melo-Martin, "Regulating Scientific Research: Should Scientists Be Left Alone?," *FASEB Journal*, March 2008. www.fasebj.org.

Chapter One: What Are the Origins of the Human Embryo Experimentation Debate?

3. Quoted in Marcia Clemmitt, "Stem Cell Research," *CQ Researcher*, September 9, 2006. www.cqresearcher.com.
4. Quoted in Genetics and Public Policy Center, "Cloning: Dickey-Wicker Amendment," 2010. www.dnapolicy.org.
5. Harold Varmus, *The Art and Politics of Science*. New York: Norton, 2009, p. 209.
6. NIH Stem Cell Information, "NIH Guidelines for Research Using Human Pluripotent Stem Cells," press release, August 23, 2000. http://stemcells.nih.gov.
7. George Bush, "President Discusses Stem Cell Research," White House, August 9, 2001. http://georgewbush-whitehouse.archives.gov.
8. Quoted in BBC News, "Bush 'Out of Touch' on Stem Cells," July 20, 2006. http://news.bbc.co.uk.
9. Quoted in Coalition for the Advancement of Medical Research, "Quotes in Support of Embryonic Stem Cell Research," 2012. www.camradvocacy.org.
10. Quoted in Steven Reinberg, "FDA OKs 1st Embryonic Stem Cell Trial," *Washington Post*, January 23, 2009. www.washingtonpost.com.
11. Quoted in Eryn Brown, "Geron Exits Stem Cell Research," *Los Angeles Times*, November 15, 2011. http://articles.latimes.com.
12. Barack Obama, "Removing Barriers to Responsible Scientific Research Involving Human Stem Cells," executive order, White House, March 9, 2009. www.whitehouse.gov.

Chapter Two: Is Human Embryo Experimentation Moral?

13. D.C. Wertz, "Embryo and Stem Cell Research in the United States: History and Politics," *Gene Therapy*, June 2002. www.ncbi.nlm.nih.gov.
14. Quoted in Gina Kolata, "Man Who Helped Start Stem Cell War May End It," *New York Times*, November 22, 2007. www.nytimes.com.

15. Quoted in American Catholic.org, "Pope John Paul II Addresses President Bush," July 23, 2001. www.americancatholic.org.

16. Quoted in Thomas A. Shannon, "Stem-Cell Research: How Catholic Ethics Guide Us," American Catholic.org. www.americancatholic.org.

17. Robert P. George and Christopher Tollefsen, *Embryo: A Defense of Human Life*. New York: Doubleday, 2008, pp. 50–51.

18. Scott Klusendorf, "Is Embryonic Stem Cell Research Morally Complex?," Life Training Institute. www.prolifetraining.com.

19. Quoted in Clemmitt, "Stem Cell Research."

20. George and Tollefsen, *Embryo*, p. 5.

21. Quoted in Clemmitt, "Stem Cell Research."

22. Quoted in Patricia Schudy, "An Embryo by Any Other Name?," *National Catholic Reporter*, August 26, 2005. http://natcath.org.

23. Ronald A. Lindsey, "Adult Reasoning About Embryos," Center for Inquiry, August 27, 2010. www.centerforinquiry.net.

24. Jane Maienschein, *Whose View of Life? Embryos, Cloning, and Stem Cells*. Cambridge, MA: Harvard University Press, 2003, pp. 261–62.

25. Bonnie Steinbock, "Why I Reject the Created/Spare Distinction," *UAlbany Magazine*, Fall 2005. www.albany.edu.

26. Steinbock, "Why I Reject the Created/Spare Distinction."

27. Stanley Fields and Mark Johnston, *Genetic Twists of Fate*. Cambridge, MA: MIT Press, 2010, p. 70.

28. Michael Kinsley, "Science Fiction: What Pro-Lifers Are Missing in the Stem-Cell Debate," *Slate*, July 7, 2006. www.slate.com.

29. Quoted in Sanford M. Goodman, "Waste of Surplus Embryos Ignores Life-Saving Potential," *Omaha World Herald*, June 18, 2010. www.omaha.com.

30. Amy Coxon, "Frozen Embryos: Stem Cell Source or Human Life?," Center for Bioethics and Human Dignity, June 2, 2005. http://cbhd.org.

31. Fields and Johnston, *Genetic Twists of Fate*, p. 69.

32. Quoted in Linda Douglass, "Abortion Foes Say Stem Cell Research Unnecessary," ABC News, April 27, 2007. http://abcnews.go.com.

33. Quoted in Maggie Fox, "Embryonic Stem Cells Made Without Embryos," ABC Science, November 21, 2007. www.abc.net.au.

34. Gene Tarne and David Prentice, "Playing Politics with Stem Cells," *American Thinker*, August 8, 2010. www.americanthinker.com.

35. Louis Guenin, "The Ethics of Human Embryonic Stem Cell Research," International Society for Stem Cell Research. www.isscr.org.

Chapter Three: Is Human Embryo Experimentation Necessary?

36. Quoted in the Coalition for the Advancement of Medical Research, "A Catalyst for Cures: Embryonic Stem Cell Research," January 12, 2009. www.camradvocacy.org.

37. Francis Collins, Hearing before a Subcommittee of the Committee on Appropriations, United States Senate, 111th Congress, September 16, 2010. www.gpo.gov.

38. Collins, Hearing before a Subcommittee of the Committee on Appropriations.

39. Coalition for the Advancement of Medical Research, "A Catalyst for Cures."

40. International Society for Stem Cell Research, "Top Ten Things to Know About Stem Cell Treatments." www.isscr.org.

41. Quoted in Reinberg, "FDA OKs 1st Embryonic Stem Cell Trial."

42. Quoted in Rob Stein, "First Hints That Stem Cells Can Help Patients Get Better," NPR, January 23, 2012. www.npr.org.

43. Quoted in Stein, "First Hints That Stem Cells Can Help Patients Get Better."

44. Quoted in Stein, "First Hints That Stem Cells Can Help Patients Get Better."

45. Quoted in Stein, "First Hints That Stem Cells Can Help Patients Get Better."

46. Quoted in Paul Recer, "Stem Cells Raise Hope for Diabetics," Associated Press, May 1, 2012. http://sci.rutgers.edu.

47. Quoted in the Coalition for the Advancement of Medical Research, "A Catalyst for Cures."

48. Quoted in Michael Fumento, "Decades Away: The Dirty Secret of Embryonic Stem Cell Research," Forbes, July 2009. www.forbes.com.

Chapter Four: What Are the Alternatives to Human Embryo Experimentation?

49. Quoted in UVA Today, "Cord Blood Stem Cell Transplants Now Available at U.Va.," March 23, 2012. www.virginia.edu.

50. Quoted in Medical News Today, "Type 1 Diabetes Reversed with Stem Cells from Cord Blood," January 11, 2012. www.medicalnewstoday.com.

51. Quoted in University of Miami Miller School of Medicine, "DRI Study Shows Stem Cells Can Replace Anti-rejection Drug for Transplants," March 20, 2012. http://med.miami.edu.

52. Quoted in BBC News, "Stem Cells Beat Kidney Rejection," BBC News, March 8, 2012. www.bbc.co.uk.

53. Jean Peduzzi-Nelson, "Testimony on the Promise of Human Stem Cell Science," testimony to the US Senate Committee on Appropriations Subcommittee on Labor, Health and Human Services, and Education," September 16, 2010. www.appropriations.senate.gov.

54. Quoted in Ron Winslow, "To Fix a Heart, Doctors Train Girl's Body to Grow New Part," Wall Street Journal, March 20, 2012. http://online.wsj.com.

55. Quoted in Winslow, "To Fix a Heart, Doctors Train Girl's Body to Grow New Part."

56. Quoted in Lorie Johnson, "Adult Stem Cells May Help Fight Heart Disease," CBN News, April 11, 2012. www.cbn.com.

57. Quoted in UC Davis Medical Center, "UC Davis Investigators Develop Method of Directing Stem Cells to Increase Bone Formation and Bone Strength," February 6, 2012. www.ucdmc.ucdavis.edu.

58. Peduzzi-Nelson, "Testimony on the Promise of Human Stem Cell Science."

59. Mary L. Davenport, "The Truth About Stem Cell Research," *American Thinker*, September 9, 2004. www.americanthinker.com.

60. International Society for Stem Cell Research, "Understanding Stem Cells." www.isscr.org.

61. Quoted in Kate Sheppard, "Komen's Position on Stem Cells Remains Unclear," *Mother Jones*, February 3, 2012. www.motherjones.com.

62. International Society for Stem Cell Research, "Understanding Stem Cells."

63. Quoted in Rick Weiss, "Scientists Cure Mice of Sickle Cell Using Stem Cell Technique," *Washington Post*, December 7, 2007. www.washington post.com.

64. Quoted in the Coalition for the Advancement of Medical Research, "A Catalyst for Cures."

65. Quoted in the Coalition for the Advancement of Medical Research, "A Catalyst for Cures."

66. International Society for Stem Cell Research, "Understanding Stem Cells."

Chapter Five: How Should Human Embryo Experimentation Be Funded?

67. Quoted in Craig Gordon, "Nancy Reagan Praises Obama," *Politico*, March 9, 2009. www.politico.com.

68. Quoted in First Read, "Reactions to Obama, Stem Cells," MSNBC.com, March 9, 2009. http://firstread.msnbc.msn.com.

69. J. Randy Forbes, "Forbes Criticizes President's Stem Cell Decision," press release, March 9, 2009. http://forbes.house.gov.

70. Orrin Hatch, "Orrin Hatch on Abortion," On the Issues. www.ontheissues .org.

71. Quoted in Aaron D. Levine, ed., *States and Stem Cells*. Princeton, NJ: Policy Research Institute for the Region, 2006. www.princeton.edu.

72. California Institute for Regenerative Medicine, "Progress Toward Therapies," 2011. www.cirm.ca.gov.

73. Quoted in Levine, *States and Stem Cells*.

74. Sigrid Fry-Revere, "Best Hope Lies in Privately Funded Stem Cell Research," Cato Institute, April 30, 2007. www.cato.org.

75. Quoted in Rob Stein, "Controversy over Stem-Cell Research Keeps Charities on Sidelines," NPR, February 7, 2012. www.npr.org.

76. Quoted in Stein, "Controversy over Stem-Cell Research Keeps Charities on Sidelines."

Related Organizations and Websites

American Association for the Advancement of Science (AAAS)
1200 New York Ave. NW
Washington, DC 20005
phone: (202) 326-6400
e-mail: webmaster@aaas.org
website: www.aaas.org

The AAAS is a global organization that seeks to advance science around the world through education, initiatives in public policy, international programs, and membership activities. To foster awareness of science and technology, the AAAS publishes and disseminates many scientific reports, books, and newsletters, as well as the journal *Science*.

American Life League
PO Box 1350
Stafford, VA 22555
phone: (540) 659-4171
fax: (540) 659-2586
website: www.all.org

The American Life League, the largest grassroots Catholic organization in the United States, is committed to the protection of all human life beginning at the moment of conception. The league believes that obtaining stem cells from an embryo is highly unethical and disseminates a wide array of information, including brochures, newsletters, and videos, to help spread their views.

Center for Bioethics and Human Dignity

Trinity International University
2065 Half Day Rd.
Deerfield, IL 60015
phone: (847) 317-8180
e-mail: info@cbhd.org
website: www.cbhd.org

The Center for Bioethics and Human Dignity explores pressing bioethical issues of the day from a Christian perspective. The center conducts research and theological analysis of bioethical topics, including the ethical issues associated with stem cell research, and provides a broad array of resources for further study.

Coalition for the Advancement of Medical Research (CAMR)

750 Seventeenth St. NW, Suite 1100
Washington, DC 20006
phone: (202) 725-0339
website: www.camradvocacy.org

The CAMR comprises one hundred nationally recognized patient organizations, universities, scientific societies, and foundations that together promote the development of treatment and cures for individuals with life-threatening illnesses. The CAMR's advocacy focuses on stem cell research, SCNT, and related research fields.

Do No Harm: The Coalition of Americans for Research Ethics

1100 H St. NW, Suite 700
Washington, DC 20005
phone: (202) 347-6840
fax: (202) 347-6849
website: www.stemcellresearch.org

Do No Harm is a coalition of scientists working to promote their view that the destruction of a human embryo in order to acquire stem cells is immoral and unnecessary. The coalition supports the use of ASCs and other alternatives to human ESC research and acts as a clearinghouse for news and information about embryonic and nonembryonic stem cell sources.

Family Research Council for Human Life and Bioethics

801 G St. NW
Washington, DC 20001
phone: (202) 393-2100
fax: (202) 393-2134
website: www.frc.org

The Family Research Council believes that life begins at conception. The council opposes abortion, euthanasia, and many forms of biotechnology, including human embryo experimentation, and promotes its views through education, outreach, and grassroots mobilization.

Hastings Center

21 Malcolm Gordon Rd.
Garrison, NY 10524
phone: (845) 424-4040
fax: (845) 424-4545
e-mail: mail@thehastingscenter.org
website: www.thehastingscenter.org

The Hastings Center is an independent, nonprofit research institute that seeks to address ethical issues in the areas of health, medicine, and the environment. The center conducts research on bioethical issues, including the use of ESC research, and collaborates with policy makers on issues that affect public policies.

International Society for Stem Cell Research (ISSCR)

111 Deer Lake Rd., Suite 100
Deerfield, IL 60015
phone: (847) 509-1944
fax: (847) 480-9282
website: www.isscr.org

The ISSCR is an independent, nonprofit organization established to promote the exchange and dissemination of information related to stem cells and to encourage research involving stem cells. The society publishes the *Pulse*, a monthly newsletter that provides the latest research news and other topical information regarding stem cell research.

National Institutes of Health (NIH) Stem Cell Information
9000 Rockville Pike
Bethesda, MD 20892
phone: (301) 496-4000
e-mail: stemcell@mail.nih.gov
website: http://stemcells.nih.gov

The NIH is a branch of the US Department of Health and Human Services. As the nation's primary medical research agency, the NIH conducts and supports research on a variety of diseases, disorders, and treatments. It is the largest source of funding for stem cell research. Its website provides abundant information on stem cell research and related topics.

WiCell Research Institute
PO Box 7365
Madison, WI 53707
phone: (888) 204-1782
e-mail: info@wicell.org
website: www.wicell.corg

WiCell Research Institute was established by the Wisconsin Alumni Research Foundation after James Thomson, a researcher at the University of Wisconsin, first established independent ESC lines. The mission of WiCell today is to support stem cell research, development, and education. WiCell maintains the National Stem Cell Bank, which supplies ESCs to researchers.

Additional Reading

Books

Brendan E. Aylesworth, *Stem Cell Research and Science: Background and Issues*. Hauppauge, NY: Nova Science, 2010.

Christian Drapeau, *Cracking the Stem Cell Code*. Portland, OR: Sutton Hart, 2010.

Courtney Farrell, *The Abortion Debate*. Edina, MN: ABDO, 2008.

Stanley Fields and Mark Johnston, *Genetic Twists of Fate*. Cambridge, MA: MIT Press, 2010.

Leo Furcht and William Hoffman, *The Stem Cell Dilemma: The Scientific Breakthroughs, Ethical Concerns, Political Tensions, and Hope Surrounding Stem Cell Research*. New York: Arcade, 2011.

Karen van Kampen, *The Golden Cell: Gene Therapy, Stem Cells and the Quest for the Next Great Medical Breakthrough*. New York: HarperCollins, 2010.

Alice Park, *The Stem Cell Hope: How Stem Cell Medicine Can Change Our Lives*. New York: Hudson Street, 2011.

Periodicals

Sarah Boseley, "Stem Cells: Great Expectations," *Guardian* (Manchester, UK), September 22, 2011.

Eryn Brown, "Stem Cells: Research Funding and the 2012 Elections," *Los Angeles Times*, November 21, 2011.

B.D. Colen, "Breakthrough in Cell Reprogramming," *Harvard Gazette*, September 30, 2010.

David Cyranoski, "Cloned Human Embryo Makes Working Stem Cells," *Nature*, October 5, 2011.

Julia Galef, "You Say Embryo, I Say Parthenote," *Scientific American*, November 4, 2011.

Leila Haghighat, "Regenerative Medicine Repairs Mice from Top to Toe," *Nature*, April 18, 2012.

Gardner Harris, "U.S. Judge Rules Against Obama's Stem Cell Policy," *New York Times*, August 23, 2010.

Bernadine Healy, "Why Embryonic Stem Cells Are Obsolete," *U.S. News & World Report*, March 4, 2009.

Jason Koebler, "Blindness Study Opens the Door for Further Stem Cell Trials," *U.S. News & World Report*, January 25, 2012.

Joanna Moorhead, "Magic Cells: Babies Who Save Lives," *Guardian* (London), March 18, 2012.

Ian Sample, "Transplanted Cells Allow Mice with Night Blindness to See in Dark," *Guardian* (London), April 18, 2012.

Stem Cell Research News, "New Stem Cell Discovery Could Spur Development of Brain Treatments," April 21, 2012.

Ann Trafton, "Stem Cells Could Drive Hepatitis Research Forward," *MIT News*, February 1, 2012.

Internet Sources

Timothy Boyer, "Will Stem Cell Retinal Transplants Cause Blindness (in Critics)?," EmaxHealth, January 23, 2012. www.emaxhealth.com/8782/will-stem-cell-retinal-transplants-cause-blindness-critics.

ScienceDaily, "Stem Cells Repair Damaged Spinal Cord Tissue," October 8, 2010. www.sciencedaily.com/releases/2010/10/101008082736.htm.

———, "Understanding the Beginnings of Embryonic Stem Cells Helps Predict the Future," October 13, 2011. www.sciencedaily.com/releases/2011/10/111013121501.htm.

Gene Tarne and David Prentice, "Playing Politics with Stem Cells," *American Thinker*, August 8, 2010. www.americanthinker.com/2010/08/playing_politics_with_stem_cel.html.

Index